Happy
Baby,
Happy
Family

Happy
Baby,
Happy
Family

Learning to
trust yourself
and enjoy
your baby

Sarah Beeson MBE

Edited by Amy Beeson

Thorsons

Thorsons
An imprint of HarperCollins*Publishers*
1 London Bridge Street
London SE1 9GF

www.harpercollins.co.uk

First published by Thorsons 2015

3 5 7 9 10 8 6 4

A catalogue record of this book is
available from the British Library

ISBN 978-0-00-752011-4

Printed and bound in Great Britain by
Clays Ltd, St Ives plc

MIX
Paper from
responsible sources
FSC **FSC** **C007454**
www.fsc.org

To my family Amy, Takbir and Ava

Contents

Preface

Sarah Beeson MBE

In our lives there are often times when we feel overwhelmed by responsibility – even when it's something we've been longing for, the reality can be a bit of a shock. When I started my nursing and health visiting career, the challenges I faced and overcame influenced the rest of my life. Becoming a parent, too, can be all-consuming and you begin to question whether you can do it. After four decades devoted to better understanding the needs of children, I can honestly say that this is the best generation of parents there has ever been.

During wonderful years nursing at Hackney Hospital I discovered that my calling was to be a health visitor, and then there was no looking back. I went on to be one of the youngest health visitors in the country, working with families in Kent and then Staffordshire. I was honoured to receive the MBE from Her Majesty Queen Elizabeth II for services to children and families. My health-prevention work was also recognised when I was given the Queen's Nursing Institute Award. Life as a health visitor was hard work, inspiring, exhausting and very fulfilling. I thought I'd continue working in the community until my retirement and then settle down to a quiet life in the country.

The inspiration for putting pen to paper on the advice I shared every day with parents as a health visitor was the arrival of my own grandchild. I had been working on how best to communicate the emotional needs of children in my everyday practice since the 1970s, but I hadn't written anything except a few articles and leaflets. At the heart of all the practical advice I was sharing was the wish to ensure parents could see *how* they were meeting their baby's emotional needs, and *why* it is so important.

Health visiting gave me the opportunity not just to help families but to learn from them. To really make a difference you have to address the needs of the whole family, and, most importantly, to listen to their problems, concerns and worries. The first step is to build a relationship with parents and earn their trust in order to give the advice that is right for them.

If you are in the UK and have a health visitor, they may be someone you have a close relationship with or it may be that due to the rapidly declining numbers of health visitors and the service being reduced, your health visitor might not play a big part of your experience with your new baby. I know there is nothing like a one-on-one service, but I do hope this book will help parents to feel like they have access to the advice I have built up over a lifetime of practice in the community.

A good health visitor doesn't think they know it all, no matter how long they've practised; when you walk into someone's home or speak to them at clinic you're just getting a glimpse of how things are. A health visitor has to give families both time and the opportunity to engage. Families shouldn't fit the health visiting service – the service offered should be shaped around the needs of families, and at some point every parent needs support, someone to talk to, advice and solutions. Every parent needs that, including me.

When you offer parenting advice, it's crucial that mums and dads don't feel judged and that you don't have a one-size-fits-all approach. When parents are talking to you, if you are thinking about what you are going to say next then you aren't really listening, and the opportunity to really help them will be missed. That has always been my approach to health visiting; it's one I learned from working with some truly exceptional nurses and health visitors right at the beginning of my career, and it has translated into the style of advice I offer to parents.

My journey from health visiting to writing started when my lovely daughter Amy Beeson became pregnant and asked me to email her advice on how to feed her baby for the first time. It was a joy to pass on all the secrets I'd learned from working with knowledgeable health professionals and dedicated parents. Amy told me she hadn't come across my style of advice in any of the baby books she was reading. There was so much she and her friends wanted to know; could I do some more? Before I knew it, I was writing a parenting book, and Amy was editing it for me during her Little One's nap times. Time flew by and my daughter's year of maternity leave was over. It's such a difficult time for so many women; few of us ever feel we've got the balance between all our responsibilities right. Then something life changing happened: not just one but several publishers wanted our parenting book (the book you're reading right now). We were thrilled, and surprised they also wanted us to write my true story of nursing in Hackney (*The New Arrival*) and about health visiting in Kent in the 1970s (*She's Arrived!*).

Amy and I waved goodbye to our steady jobs and now work together writing and meeting wonderful readers and parents. I never imagined I'd be an author but, more importantly, passing on my knowledge and experience to parents is a huge privilege – and sometimes it's a little daunting. Focusing on why I do the job that I do is what really matters, and it's no different today than it was all those years ago. I want a world filled with happy babies, and for mums and dads to see what a fantastic start in life they are giving their children by putting them at the centre of their lives and meeting their emotional needs as well as their practical ones.

I hope your own new arrival fills your life with joy – and thank you for letting us come on this special journey with you.

Visit www.sarahbeeson.org to find out more and download your FREE poo colour chart.

Discovering Your Parenting Style

One thing I've learned after four decades working with literally thousands of families from all walks of life and in all kinds of circumstances is this – there isn't one perfect way of parenting; every single baby and family is unique. It is the parents or the person who is the main carer for a child who has the greatest insight into the needs of their Little One.

I promise you, no matter who you are or how things might look from the outside, every good parent has doubts about their abilities or the choices they are making. One way you could use this book is as a companion that offers solutions to help you find your parenting style and to give you reassurance when you need it, so you can be the parent you want to be. Feeling confident, authentic and positive about your role as a parent is key to building a loving relationship with your child. If there is one thing I'd like this book to achieve, it would be to help parents trust themselves and enjoy their time with their baby, because they grow so fast.

I have a simple philosophy underlying all my parenting advice: babies who have a strong attachment to their mothers (or the main caregiver) are more likely to grow into happy children, adolescents and adults who have a good relationship with you and will turn to you in times of need and celebrate with you in times of joy. It sounds simplistic but I do believe that when parents love and nurture their children the result is a happy baby, as well as happy mums and dads; and ultimately this results in happier families and a better society.

In this book we'll look at practical care from birth until your baby's first birthday. At first life will revolve around feeding, trying to get them to sleep and an endless stream of dirty nappies, but things do change rapidly during your baby's first year. Experience has shown me that it is helpful for mums and dads to know what to expect and to have some solutions for dealing with common problems. We'll look at what it means when a baby is behaving in a certain way, what you can do to help your baby, and how the approach you take will reinforce your Little One's ever-growing sense of attachment to you.

The one-to-one service I offered as a health visitor cannot be fully replicated in this book, as so much comes out of having an ongoing conversation with mums and dads. I don't think there has ever been a single mum who would have received all the advice that's in here, because she wouldn't have needed it. It is unrealistic and unhelpful to suggest there is one way of caring for a baby. To create the expectation that there is a single right way of doing things doesn't help parents, and it doesn't help babies – it just makes people feel angry or anxious.

Many parents want to learn more about their child's development and the practical and emotional needs of their baby – but where do you start? There is so much information but often it doesn't go into the detail you may need, and you aren't always sure of the authority of the person who's written it. When it comes to childcare, advice can be very slanted to a particular method of caring for babies, and you may feel that you and your baby don't fit that mould. We have to experiment and do what works for us and our family.

The unconditional and overwhelming love most parents have for their baby is like no other (though not everyone will experience that right away; for some it takes time and can depend on the circumstances around the birth of their child). It is love that can give you an inner strength you never knew you had. Love is the greatest gift we can ever give our children; a baby that feels loved every day is going to be a happy baby.

We feel loved when our needs are met, when we get daily affection and understanding, when we are treated with kindness and respect, and are secure and know we come first. A baby is no different; they are just a tiny person who needs that love more than anything – a baby needs to know there is at least one person who absolutely cares for them. Everything else you do is a choice; we make small decisions every day and are continually adapting to new situations – that is the most any parent can do.

It's good to understand what your baby's needs are and base your day around them, but you'll probably need some flexibility to adapt to what each day brings. You'll notice patterns emerging and develop a rhythm and understanding of what makes your baby happy so you can create an adaptable mini-routine that is right for you both. It's paramount that you give yourself the time and space to develop confidence in yourself as a parent and recognise your ability to tune in to your baby's daily needs. How you want to care for your baby and shape your day is down to you; every family is different, and your baby is a unique individual, but there are basic needs that all babies have, and it can only boost your confidence and ability as a parent to read, think and discuss what they are.

For me the Dalai Lama expresses this perfectly: he says, 'Everyone can understand from natural experience and common sense that affection is crucial from the day of birth; it is the basis of life.' Keep that in mind and you are already on the road to forming a wonderful relationship with your baby.

I hope you enjoy your baby every step of the way, and remember there's no better or more challenging role in the world than becoming a parent. I know how much you want to do the best you can for your baby, and I've seen first hand that more and more parents are making their baby their top priority – and it's having a big effect: happier babies.

1

Every Day You Breastfeed Is a Huge Achievement

If you choose to breastfeed it will have lots of benefits for both you and your baby. Give it a go if you can and want to, would be my advice, but don't be pressured in any way. This is your baby and your decision; no one should make you feel guilty about your choice to breastfeed or not. Take it one day at a time – understanding breastfeeding and having realistic expectations of yourself and your baby will make it more likely you'll be relaxed and have a positive experience.

Breastfeeding is a wonderful thing; there are huge health benefits for mother and child, and it helps to develop attachment – but it's not always easy. Please don't think you are doing something wrong if you find it challenging, because it can be. You wouldn't expect to get into a car for the first time and just drive it; it takes practice and then one day you find yourself driving along without really even having to think about it.

Nearly all babies have some frustration when learning how to feed; you're *both* doing something new for the first time, and practice makes perfect when it comes to breastfeeding.

The first time you breastfeed

If possible, put your baby to the breast as soon as possible after delivery so they benefit from the colostrum (the milk you produce from birth) – it's full of antibodies and nutrients that are perfect for your baby.

Making Milk for Your Baby

The milk you produce after giving birth is called **colostrum** – it is designed by nature especially for your baby to help them fight infection and get off to a flying start. It is thick, yellow and chock-full of protective antibodies.

There are three stages of milk production during the first week:

1st Stage   Colostrum produced from birth to 3–4 days
2nd Stage   Transitional milk from 3–4 days to 7+ days
3rd Stage   Mature milk from 7+ days

Skin to skin

Put your naked baby (with or without nappy) against your bare chest or tummy and hold them close. Relax and enjoy your baby – you've been waiting for this moment. Skin-to-skin contact as soon as possible after birth is beneficial for babies, mums and dads – it is a very special feeling.

Skin to skin helps to stimulate your body's production of breast milk and allows both parents to bond with their baby. Most hospitals encourage skin to skin and will help you do it for the first time as soon as your baby is born. It will help your Little One (I'll refer to your baby as 'LO' throughout this book!) to feel comforted and secure.

Visualising holding your baby for the first time is a positive image many women use during labour to help them focus on the end result. You can go back to skin to skin over the weeks and months to come when your baby needs comforting – babies just adore it.

Breastfeeding if your baby is in a special care baby unit

Some babies, due to complications or premature birth, need extra care in a neonatal unit from dedicated hospital staff. I know how this feels: my own baby, Amy, was seven weeks premature and weighed only 2 lb 11 oz and was in the incubator for five weeks. You may feel a mixture of anxiety, hope, love, fear and anger that this is happening to you and your baby. Many women find the separation from their baby overwhelming, and naturally so. Like any new mum, taking care of yourself will help you to give your child the love and care they need. In the days, weeks and months to come, it may be you can easily put it behind you, but some mums do find the experience can be difficult to shake off. (If you find you are still feeling anxious or low about the experience you had giving birth, have a look at Chapter 4, Being a New Mum Is Life Changing).

If your baby is in an incubator or needs special care, it is still possible to breastfeed. All babies benefit from breast milk, but poorly or premature babies really do – your milk will help give your Little One the nourishment they need. It might be that you need to express your breast milk rather than feed directly from the breast (have a look at the section on expressing breast milk later in this chapter, page 29). You may only be able to express a little milk during the first few days, but that precious colostrum is going to make a big difference to your baby and it is full of antibodies. Both you and the nursing and midwifery team may feed your baby through a tube until the baby is ready to feed independently at the breast.

As soon as a newborn baby shows they are ready to suckle and are more alert you should be able to start breastfeeding your baby whilst you're in hospital. If you're on a separate ward or have been discharged you can leave expressed breast milk for the times you won't be there.

It is the skin-to-skin contact that will help stimulate the milk supply and give you the opportunity to have some one-to-one time with your Little One. Enjoy those cuddles and remember, the more contact you have, the better. It'll help you relax and become more familiar with each other, and will get your baby demanding and you supplying breast milk.

It's likely you will be offered professional help to get you started with breastfeeding, but this is no reflection on you – breastfeeding in these circumstances is challenging. Getting the right support, whether that's from the nursing and midwifery team, family or friends, will make a big difference – you are not alone, take it one step at a time.

How breastfeeding supports attachment between mother and baby

The touch of your skin your baby experiences during breast-feeding, the sound of your breath and heartbeat all contribute towards the development of a very strong bond between mother and child. Breastfeeding mums have to put their baby at the centre of their lives. You cannot leave your baby for long periods of time if you are breastfeeding, so, without giving it much conscious thought, you will naturally be tuning in to the rhythm of your baby, instinctively putting their needs first and doing all the elementary things that help to build strong attachment. You'll be enjoying the looks, smiles and little touches your baby only gives you whilst you're nursing. You'll hear their first coos and gurgles and have plenty of opportunity to talk, sing to and cuddle your baby. All of this will help your Little One to feel loved and secure, because the foundation of attachment is laid down from the earliest days of your baby's life.

Developing your latching technique

During the first week, when the milk comes in, sometimes women experience a toe-curling sensation for the first few seconds as the baby latches on (but this won't last much beyond the first week). This sensation varies from woman to woman – for some it's a small sharp shock, for others it's akin

Trust Yourself

Getting Your LO to Open Wide

Brush your baby's top lip and/or cheek with your nipple. This makes them open nice and wide for the whole areola.

to plucking your eyebrows, and then there are those fortunate mums who don't feel a thing.

As long as your baby is properly attached, any discomfort should last for only a few moments. If pain persists during the feed, I'd suggest talking to a health professional about latching on and positions, to find a solution that's going to be right for you.

Start by supporting your baby's head, shoulders, neck and back. Tilt your baby's head back safely to bring them up towards the breast. Your baby needs to have a big open mouth and be brought up towards the nipple from underneath the breast to enable them to latch on.

You need to get the whole areola (the dark circle surrounding the nipple) or nearly all of it into the baby's mouth to ensure good attachment. Your baby's nose should be in line with your nipple, with their chin touching your breast, keeping the baby's nose clear so as not to obstruct breathing.

For most women breastfeeding is a big challenge, though a very rewarding one. It is demanding both in the time it takes and in the levels of energy it uses. There will be the occasional woman who never has a day's difficulty, but most women have issues at some point – but all problems have solutions and you'll be so pleased you kept on going.

Keeping the Nose Free

Help to keep the nose clear from the breast by drawing your baby's hips and bottom towards you at a slightly tilted angle. LO's body will be in a straight line but the head is tilted up towards you so you can look into their eyes.

The Latching Technique

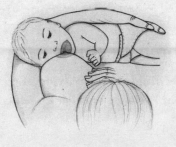

1 Get the baby's body in a straight line and lift the baby up to the breast from below.

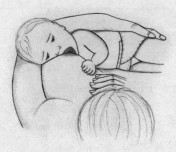

2 Line up your baby's nose to the nipple.

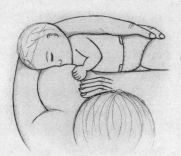

3 Get as much of the dark nipple area as possible into the baby's mouth, still keeping the nose clear.

I always say that every day you breastfeed is a massive achievement, so just take it one day at a time. Using a relaxation technique that might have helped you in labour could help you get through those first few uncomfortable seconds. Just do what feels right for you.

Top three secrets of breastfeeding

The secrets of getting breastfeeding off to a flying start – remember the three Ps: Position, Patience and Perseverance.

1. Get in a comfortable position

Many babies thrash about, moving from side to side, missing the nipple completely and getting very annoyed. This is perfectly normal and no failing on your part; just be patient and keep on trying. If you watch any baby animal feeding for the first time on nature programmes, they always do this, pummelling and bumping into their mum. This is nature's way of helping the milk let down so you produce more milk. It is supply and demand – and it can be difficult to believe just how much milk

Trust Yourself

Get Comfy

Feeding takes time, so make the most of it. Get yourself set up with a drink, a snack, the remote control, and your phone or an eBook all within reach. Place one comfy cushion behind your back, and a cushion to support the baby as well if you want to, and put your feet up – when else will you get the chance!

Happy Baby Breastfeeding Positions

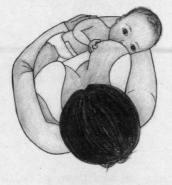

Cradle or cross-cradle

Place the baby's head in the crook of the supporting arm and hold the baby across your body with either the same arm or both arms.

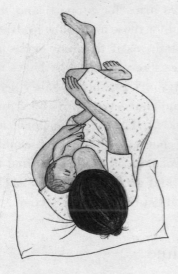

Side-lying

Support the baby's head in the crook of the arm on your side, resting the baby's body against your upper body.

a newborn baby demands. The more the baby suckles, the more milk you will produce, and you'll notice they often place a little hand on your breast or tap it; they are instinctively doing this to let the milk down.

Mastering the technique of breastfeeding is simply getting into the right position so your baby can swallow easily. That's why

having the baby in a straight line enables them to do this. Two positions most mothers use are the cradle and cross-cradle (using either one or two arms for support) and the side-lying position (really useful for those night-time feeds).

Positioning is really important, as if the baby sucks on the end of the nipple it becomes sore very quickly. That's no fun for baby or mum, as they won't get the feed they need and you will be in pain and find your levels of tiredness and frustration escalate very quickly. (If this does happen, all is not lost; later on in this chapter we'll look at coping strategies if you experience problems, allowing you time to heal, give the baby their feed, and get things back on track. You can also look up problems quickly in the A–Z section.)

2. Be patient; it takes time

Nearly all babies (and many mums) have some frustration when starting to feed. Women are often disappointed or reproach themselves if they don't take to breastfeeding instantly, and think they are doing something wrong. I've heard many a woman say, 'They never said it was going to be difficult in the antenatal classes. What am I doing wrong?' You are doing nothing wrong, you are giving your all, and the fact you are breastfeeding is amazing. Focus on getting yourself something to eat, a wash

and your head down for a nap when you can, because there won't be time for anything else in the early days. If you'd never used a computer or played an instrument, no one would expect you to do it perfectly on the first day, not even in the first week.

Also let's not forget your body has just done something miraculous – you've given birth! You're tired and life is never going to be the same again – emotions run high – one minute you'll feel on top of the world and the next you can feel like you want to run in the bathroom and lock the door for 5 minutes' peace. Staying calm, taking a deep breath and taking your time to get into the right position are what's needed.

You both need support and the opportunity to get used to feeding, and in the early days it takes a lot of concentration and energy. I've known women who've needed complete silence and have banned the television being on whilst learning to breastfeed, or others who have needed the TV or radio on to distract them and help pass the time. Some women find at first they can only feed in bed and don't want lots of clothes getting in the way; others like to rest the baby on a pillow in their laps; some want to be lying down – just do whatever feels right for you.

Be patient with yourself and your baby, and be flexible, as your baby's needs and your ability to interpret those needs will change and develop with each feed. Each day you feed, you'll grow in confidence, improve your technique and find a range of different positions and methods that work for you. Soon you *will* be able to pop them on whenever and wherever you need to with ease. Even when you're proficient at breastfeeding, everyone has the odd difficult day; when that happens put it behind you and remind yourself how much you've achieved and take it one feed at a time.

3. Persevere: take it a one feed at a time

Babies can be very demanding and all-consuming. In the early days when you've had hardly any sleep, you've got sore nipples and you can't remember the last time you washed your hair, it does require great determination and perseverance to keep on going with breastfeeding – but it does get better, and you'll feel such a strong bond with your baby for doing it.

The support network you have can really make all the difference in helping you to keep on breastfeeding for as long as you want to. It may only be you that can feed the baby, but your partner and family have a big supportive role to play here, too.

It's important to ask for help and support; if you are talking to a health professional never feel that a question is silly or insignificant – it's not. In some areas other mothers who are breastfeeding or have recently breastfed their babies offer mum-to-mum support. This gives you the opportunity to get help, tips and encouragement from other mums who've had similar experiences. It can be really good to find out about nice cafés and places to go where women enjoy breastfeeding their babies, because you won't want to stay at home forever, and it's important you find places where you feel comfortable. Breastfeeding in public can be a very liberating experience – it is what breasts are for, after all!

Trust Yourself

It's Good to Talk

A problem shared really can be a problem halved. Whether it's with a professional, your mum, your sister, your partner or a friend who is going through the same thing ... breastfeeding is not without its drama days, and it's nice to know you're not the only one.

I remember when ... I first worked in rural Kent getting a desperate call from a mum late one Christmas Eve. She was near to giving up breastfeeding her newborn baby, and there was no way I was going to make her wait for help until after Boxing Day. It was getting dark and I made my way through the snow down the country lanes in my trusty Mini to see her. When I got there I saw straight away that she had a very long baby who was also a very cross baby who needed more breast milk to satisfy his mighty appetite. When I looked in his nappy he had a light green poo that only stained his terry towelling nappy. We both knew he needed more milk. I sat down with his mum and together we calmly revisited latching on and how to calm him; we talked about and tried to find a good feeding position for her, and I told her about the ways you can tell if your baby is getting enough milk. This lovely mum also needed a little TLC herself; she was rushed off her feet and needed to take a little time to eat and drink while I had a cuddle with the baby. I was with them for a couple of hours, and when I got back to my Mini I realised I'd left the headlights on and the battery was flat. Now, the snow was falling heavily and I was miles from home. I walked to the telephone box to call out the local mechanic, trying to work out how I was going to pay the bill. He came out on Christmas Eve and got my little Mini going, and when I asked him how much, he said, 'No charge, Nurse.' I learned that day that patience and perseverance are just what mums and newly qualified health visitors need to get them through. I'll never forget the kindness of that mechanic; he had the true spirit of Christmas.

Is my baby getting enough milk?

I don't think I have ever met a breastfeeding mother who didn't have some anxiety about whether her baby was getting enough milk, even when it feels like you are feeding non-stop. I have found there are three signs that tell you if a baby is getting enough milk, which I will talk you through in a moment.

I know it can be hard to believe that all your baby's food and drink needs can be satisfied by breast milk – but for the first few months they really are. It is supply and demand; the more the baby suckles, the more milk is produced, and this is why your Little One needs to feed so frequently. You'll notice your appetite increases, too, and you need to eat well and drink lots of extra fluids to make that milk.

The three signs your baby is getting enough breast milk

1st sign: the sound your baby makes when feeding

When a baby is getting mouthfuls of feed and swallowing it sounds like gulping, there will be a *glug, glug, glug* noise as the milk goes down into their stomach, often with a *siss, siss, siss* sound as well.

When the baby latches on they will feed for a few minutes and then have a little rest and a breather whilst more milk travels down. After a couple of minutes' rest, if you gently move your baby they will start up again and have some more. They may do this several times before they have finished on that breast. It's like they are saying to you, 'Not finished yet,

Mum. A little more, please.'
They will do this four or
five times before they allow
you to finish on that side,
and they will look sleepy –
milk drunk, in fact.

If you think about the
way you eat, generally we
don't take everything on our
plate in one go. Sometimes
you feel like a light lunch
and other times you fancy a

really big dinner, but you like to have a little pause in between
your starter and your main course. You'll find your baby will
have different requirements with each feed; just tune in to
them and they'll soon show you the way.

Feeding from both sides

You'll want your baby to empty the breast and get the lovely
rich hind milk that comes down towards the end of the feed.
Babies often know they have had the lot before you do, and
start crying for more and getting very cross with the empty
breast. You'll soon learn when the breast is empty, although
you may not feel any sensation as strong as you do when the
breast feels full. It can be frustrating for your baby if they
are sucking on an empty breast. Giving them the other side
as well will keep your Little One topped up and give you a
little more time in-between feeds, as the baby will be fuller
for longer.

Some babies may have both sides at most of their feeds,
others only when they are extra hungry like after a long sleep.
Sometimes it seems like they can hardly wait five seconds

while you switch them over from one breast to the other. If you've got a baby that usually just wants to feed, feed, feed with virtually no stopping, change their nappy at the start of the feed; if they are on the sleepy side, changing their nappy at 'half time' will wake them up a bit and stimulate their appetite for the other side, ensuring they get plenty of milk and a nice full tummy. Always start the next feed on the side they didn't have or that you finished on.

2nd sign: understanding how your baby gains weight

A baby's weight is individual to that baby, and comparing it to another child is not an indicator of how well they are doing – you wouldn't expect all adults to be the same height and weight. Understanding the weight gain that is right for and unique to your baby can be really helpful and put your mind at rest.

The weight your baby puts on will help you to tell if your baby is getting enough milk. If you're in the UK, the midwife and then your health visitor will weigh the baby to monitor their growth, and chart it on what is called a percentile chart (usually referred to as 'centiles'). These graphs are next to the weight pages in your Parent Held Record (The Red Book) and show how your baby is progressing along their own line.

It can be difficult to get your head round what the centiles mean. If you think about 100 babies born on the same day as your baby, they will be charted somewhere on the graph. Let's say your Little One is on the ninth centile, which means 91 babies would weigh more and eight babies less than your baby. If your baby was born on the 50th centile, half of the 100 will weigh more and half less. It doesn't matter where on the chart your baby starts; it's the progress they make along their own line that matters, not what anyone else's baby weighs. What you want to see is your baby progressing along their line or moving above it. If your baby started to drop significantly below their own centile line, you would want to get them checked and discuss why that may be happening.

Babies seem to have an inner clock that regulates how much they need to feed. Sometimes they feed very frequently and other times they can go longer and seem to be less frantic. It is amazing, but more often than not a baby follows their centile line perfectly (though if they are poorly they might deviate from their usual rate of growth until they get better). It is always good to see their progress and to act on anything that is not expected.

Your health visitor should monitor their progress with you, so keep an eye on it but don't worry about small fluctuations. If you do have any concerns about weight gain, seek help from your health visitor or doctor. Get your baby's weight checked at clinic every two weeks until you are happy with their weight gain, and then go every three to four weeks just to get it checked if you want to.

The minimum weight you would expect a breastfed baby to gain in a week would be 3–4 oz/90–120 g. Your baby may gain a lot more than this, and some babies put on 8 oz/250 g in just over a week. This is just a very rough guide, and if your baby is feeding well and having lots of wet and dirty nappies, and is content as well as looking well and active, they will be putting on the weight they need in nearly all cases.

So many women have told me they feel under pressure when their baby is losing weight in the first week. This is often due to the passing of meconium stools (the blackish first stools the baby passes after birth) and because your baby has not started to gain weight yet. If your Little One is on the large side you may find it will take them longer to regain their birth weight.

Most babies will lose some weight because they suddenly have to work very hard to get their grub; when they were a foetus, life was so easy and comfortable. Now they've got feeding, pooing and producing lots of wind to do, all of which requires a lot of effort on their part – it's no wonder they get grumpy.

How much your baby weighs can be a great source of anxiety for some mothers; it seems to be the one question people keep asking, often followed by, 'That's not much,' or 'What a whopper. What are you feeding them?' The pressure for babies to gain weight from family and friends can seem to dominate those early visits, but it is only one indicator of how well a baby is feeding. For instance, long babies or very active babies might put less weight on. Both small and big babies get a lot of weight-related comments, and mums sometimes feel that their Little One doesn't weigh enough or needs to lose weight.

If your baby is still having lots of wet and dirty nappies and is feeding well and is content, it is fine to let them go at their own pace – they'll gain in the time that is right for them, and sometimes it is unreasonable to expect them to do this in the immediate postnatal period. Some babies take up to two weeks to regain their birth weight, but if your baby is not keen to suckle and not feeding well, then get them checked at the doctor's in case jaundice is making your baby sleepy and is affecting their intake of milk.

Mostly, with perseverance and patience they will start to put weight on – then keeping pace with their appetite will be your next challenge! Don't forget: if they are weighed with a full tummy, having just fed and not having pooed yet, they will weigh a little more than a baby who has filled their nappy and is waiting for a feed.

3rd sign: lots of dirty nappies

Well-fed babies produce lots of dirty nappies. Monitor the frequency, quantity and colour of nappies – if lots of brimming mustard-coloured nappies are coming your way, you can be confident that your baby is getting enough to eat.

The first poos a baby does are the meconium stools which usually last for about three days or so. Usually on the third or fourth day this poo will change to a lighter colour with a more greenish look. Babies also get lots of wind passing through them at both ends. When your baby is past the fourth or fifth day they will do about two or more poos every day, usually just small amounts to start.

Your baby will wet and fill most nappies in the early weeks, and the stools are often very soft liquid and bright yellow like the colour of mustard. They can be frothy as well and shoot out onto the changing mat, all of which is normal (watch out for those exploding nappies!). Yellow poos tell us the baby is getting all the milk they need including the rich hind milk, which is responsible for that golden colour, and it is reassuring to know your baby is emptying the breast to get it. So, changing lots of nappies is a good thing – I promise.

The number of dirty nappies is important because if your baby weren't getting enough milk you'd notice a light green stool that would only stain the nappy, as there wouldn't be enough poo to fill it up. To get a baby back on track, more frequent feeds are needed – and if they were only taking one side, now is the time to ensure your baby feeds from both breasts at most feeds.

Darker grey/green with yellow poos do sometimes occur when the baby is a bit older – this is not a problem. The poo looks a bit mixed, somewhere between green and yellow, and can resemble little grains like rice. Some mums say this looks like tiny leaves. This poo is not a hunger stool and is fine.

Change Bag Essentials

Nipple gel
Breastfeeding pads
Shawl
Bottle of water for you
Travel pillow
Muslin
Nappies
Wipes
Nappy bags
Spare set of baby clothes

Older babies often poo less

In the early days there is an endless stream of dirty nappies, but as your baby gets older you may notice they don't do as many poos in a day, and then just poo every other day. It can often be they do three to five dirty nappies a day for a few weeks, then it goes down to two or three a day, and by 12–14 weeks some babies only do one dirty nappy a day, or even go several days without one (though some babies will always do several poos a day – just to keep you on your toes).

At this stage if there are still lots of wet nappies to change, you'll know everything is normal and your baby is being very efficient with the digestion of the milk and making fewer waste products. It may seem alarming that a baby does this, but it is normal in a fully breastfed baby before they are weaned onto solid foods.

This often happens from 10–12 weeks and in other babies at 16–20 weeks. Just be prepared that when they don't go for a little while, when they go, they really go! If you are out and about, have plenty of spare nappies, wipes and a clean set of clothes – nearly all mums experience their baby's poo explosion just at the most inconvenient moment. Every baby should produce lots of wet nappies a day – if your Little One does not have several wet nappies, or if the wee looks dark, do go and see your doctor or a health professional to see if there is a problem.

How often should I feed my baby?

This is another question new mums have a lot of anxiety over, and understandably so. The health and well-being of your baby is a big responsibility, and you want to feel confident about the choices you make about how best to care for your baby. Getting the feeding right is where it all starts, so it's good you are asking yourself this question – now here's the information you need to put your mind at rest that you are doing a great job.

It is normal for a newborn baby to feed every two to three hours (timing it from when you started the feed, not when you finished it). Your new baby's little stomach is the same size as their clenched fist, so they can only comfortably hold a small amount of milk in their tummy and then they will be ready for more – they really do need to feed that often.

Your baby is driven by an inner clock that demands food and cannot wait – they will scream, suck their fingers and work themselves up into a frenzy when they get hungry. All the while you have to get yourself a drink, go to the loo and get ready to feed again. Understandably it can be difficult to feel relaxed, but do take those few minutes you need to get ready before you start the feed, and then you'll be in a better position to feed your baby for as long as they want and as often as they want. If your baby is crying while you are getting ready to feed, ask your partner, a relative or a friend to help calm the baby using the Up-Down Technique (see Chapter 3, Sleep, Calming and Creating Your Own Routine). The calmer the baby is, the more likely they are to latch on with ease.

The gap between feeds will get longer as the weeks and months go by, and your baby will become more efficient at getting the milk they need. It can be helpful for you and your family to acknowledge to yourselves that your baby cannot practise patience but you all can. When your baby gets upset it is not that they don't like you or you are not doing a good job – just that your Little One can only focus on getting their own needs met and isn't aware that you need to eat, drink, wash and sleep as well.

This demanding time is temporary, and in retrospect you'll feel like it went by in a flash, though at the time when you are sleep-deprived and exhausted it may not feel that way. That's why reminding yourself regularly of all you've achieved – bringing your baby into the world and sustaining them completely by the milk you give them is simply amazing. Recognising the wonderful, positive things you are doing for your child and family will increase your ability to cope and increase your own sense of well-being. It'll be even better if your partner, family and friends tell you what a great mum you are, too (hint, hint).

As time goes by your confidence in your ability to interpret your baby's needs will grow. As you get more practice at caring for your baby it will become a little easier day by day, and you'll feel less anxious about getting things right and be more able to go with the flow. I believe knowing what to expect and shaping your day around the needs of your baby is a really good thing. You may hear people talk a lot about routines – though in my experience tiny babies do not have a strict routine, they don't follow a timetable. After all, each child is unique – and though there are definitely general practices we can follow, they have to be shaped around that child and their family.

You will probably start to notice patterns developing and have a mini-routine going for about a week, and then things will change again (have a look at the adaptable mini-routines in Chapter 3). Many mothers find that a baby does not behave exactly the same two days in a row, so I think the secret to success is anticipating your baby's needs but having enough flexibility to enjoy each day with your baby. Having too strict a structure can make mothers feel trapped, and that's not good for them or their Little One.

Nap times and feed times will vary, but *you can* exercise influence over your day. You and your baby will develop a rhythm that helps you read them more easily so you can pick up on the cues that tell you they're getting tired or hungry, and act on them before things escalate and tears appear. This is your baby and your life, so do what works for you. As long as your baby's needs are met, all will be well.

Is it normal for me to be this hungry?

If you are breastfeeding, yes it is! You are very likely to have a much bigger appetite than usual when you start breast-feeding – you do need to eat (you can't breastfeed a baby successfully on a salad and a crispbread). Many women crave carbohydrates, chocolate and sweet things because you need a good intake of carbohydrates to make that milk. You'll want to balance this out with a good helping of protein-rich foods and adequate fats, plus plenty of fruits and vegetables each day.

In order to make rich, plentiful breast milk, eat at least three portions of carbohydrate a day. Healthy choices are cereals, oats, bread, potatoes, rice and pasta – they are all a good source of carbohydrate as part of a balanced diet.

Never try to diet when breastfeeding, as you need your calories from a wide range of foods for nutrients (particularly no-carb or very low-carb regimes are no good for milk production). This is because breast milk has a high proportion of carbohydrate (if your milk leaks you'll see that when it dries it starches your clothing, which shows the sugar levels in the breast milk made by a good intake of carbohydrate).

Eat the foods you want and like, and only avoid foods if you think they are upsetting you or the baby. Tastes do change during pregnancy and during breastfeeding, so it may be you can no longer stomach that old favourite but you are craving things you didn't like before. Many women find they can't eat certain foods whilst breastfeeding, and if you notice your baby is very grumpy and difficult to settle or satisfy all of a sudden, look back over the past 24 hours to see if you've eaten or drunk something that might have disagreed with them. It may be that some foods that are high in fibre like bran or new potatoes, or too many fresh berries or fruit juice may upset the breast milk. It may also change your LO's poos, but this can be difficult to detect as normal poo is runny and explosive anyway.

I remember when ... my daughter Amy had just had her baby and I was staying with them to help out for the first couple of weeks. Baby Ava would feed all night long, and I used to bring Amy tea and toast in the middle of the night as it was feed, feed, feed and she needed to eat and drink enough to keep on going. I would often sit up and chat and laugh with her till the sun came up to help Amy make it through those long nights, and then once the baby had finally had enough (at about breakfast time) I used to make Amy some breakfast, and then look after the baby while she got a few hours' much-needed sleep.

Solutions to common breastfeeding problems

Sore nipples

Having sore or painful nipples is probably the most frequently experienced problem women have when breastfeeding. In the first week it can be the result of your baby first learning to feed and your milk coming in, and it can be a toe-curling experience.

When your baby first starts to suck it may be painful for the first few seconds. If the pain persists, check the position of your baby – they may be sucking on the end of the nipple and not getting the big mouthful of breast they get when correctly attached (revisit the Latching Technique section at the beginning of this chapter). If this happens, slip your little finger in at the corner of their mouth and break the suction. Adjust your position and try using a pillow if you want to (even if you are out and about, there are little travel cushions you can slip into the change bag to make life easier when feeding in public). Raise the baby up and bring them up to the breast. Check they are nose to nipple and ensure they have an open mouth coming from below the breast to latch on, getting as much of the brown area of the nipple into their mouth

Trust Yourself

Aching Back? Maybe You Need a Bigger Bra

The size of your breasts increases as the milk comes in, and many women go up several cup sizes. Having an ill-fitting bra can cause backache. A loose-fitting bra to begin with for your hospital bag and wearing around the house is fine until you feel like a trip out to get properly fitted.

as possible and having a good seal, not a 'gappy' one, and keeping the nose clear from obstruction.

When they have finished, squeeze out some hind milk and gently rub it into the nipple to help soothe and protect it. Using breastfeeding gels before and after feeding may also help make you more comfortable. Also, don't over-wash the breasts as this may actually be a cause of soreness.

Cracked nipples

If your nipples are very sore and using expressed breast milk or gel is not sufficient, then you may need to get a prescription for cream to heal the nipples. Any cream you use will need to be washed off before feeding the baby so they are fiddly and more time-consuming than using gel or hind milk. But sometimes if you use a cream for just 24 hours and let plenty of air get to the breasts, the nipple will heal a lot faster.

If you are suffering, using a cream to heal faster is well worth the bother, and much better in the long run than feeding on a very sore breast. Apply the cream in a thick layer, then wipe off with damp cotton wool before you feed your baby. I know this can be a real pain during night feeds, but do make sure it's all gone, as the baby should not ingest any of the cream.

While the nipple is healing you may want to breastfeed on only one side and express milk from the sore breast, just until it is comfortable to feed again.

If you are diagnosed with thrush, then not only will you need to finish any course of treatment to clear the infection but the baby will need to take oral medication as well (see also the A–Z section for more about thrush).

Blocked ducts

You may notice a small tender lump in your breast that could indicate a blocked duct. Try massaging the breast or using the warmth from a covered hot water bottle or warmed pad to help to disperse it. You may find this works best if you gently massage the breast to unblock the duct while you are in the bath or shower. This is best done after a feed; a good feed will help to empty the affected breast and clear the blockage. If a blocked duct does not clear it may lead to mastitis, so ask your health visitor or doctor for further advice at the earliest opportunity.

Mastitis

Mastitis can be a mild or severe inflammation of the breast and sometimes can cause fever and vomiting. If the breasts are painful and swollen and/or hot and red, you may have mastitis. Seek medical advice as soon as you notice the symptoms, especially if you have flu-like symptoms and are feeling hot and cold with achy joints and feeling generally unwell. Your doctor may prescribe some antibiotics if the mastitis has become infected. Only take medication as instructed by your health practitioner.

Drink lots of fluids and try using warm packs, or sometimes an ice pack can help, or even a small quantity of frozen peas in a plastic bag wrapped in a clean towel (remember not to eat the peas later on, though you could label them and refreeze for medicinal use again).

Do keep feeding the baby if you can, and check the position for breastfeeding and how the baby latches on to ensure you're going to be as comfortable as possible. (Revisit the Latching Techniques and positioning advice earlier in this chapter to double-check.)

Expressing breast milk (EBM)

You can express breast milk either by hand or by using a hand or electric pump so that your baby can get their milk from a sterilised bottle, cup or spoon rather than at the breast for a feed.

It is usually preferable to feed your baby at the breast and not to express milk in the early days but it may be something you want to do for a short time if you are experiencing sore nipples or you are separated from your baby. You may not be able to meet all your baby's milk needs through EBM alone but it can be a useful supplement alongside breastfeeding or for babies who are in a special care baby unit.

Breastfeeding Shopping List

Breast pads
Nipple gel or cream
Freezer bags
Steriliser
Breast pump
Bottles
Bottle brush
Nipple shields
Breastfeeding tops, dresses, cardigans
A shawl
Feeding pillow
Muslin

Breastfed babies need to get milk from both breasts as often as possible to establish and increase the supply of breast milk with frequent sucking. It is very unlikely that a mother can express the same amount of milk for her baby that feeding at the breast delivers, so unless there are special circumstances, like the baby being in a special care unit, I would advise that you feed from the breasts for the first two weeks or so to get the milk supply established.

If a baby is premature or poorly and is in a special care unit, a mum has no other choice than to use EBM if they are not allowed to put the baby to the breast. Whatever your circumstances are, expressing breast milk is hard work. It often gives you flexibility, but some women find it draining, and you will need even more sustenance to both express and also breastfeed.

EBM can be really handy to have in the fridge when your baby is demanding huge amounts of milk in the night; giving your breasts a rest, and if your partner takes over it'll give you a rest, too. Expressing milk does mean extra washing and sterilising of bottles and equipment (this is often a good job for your partner to take on; have a look at Chapter 2 to find out how to sterilise bottles and equipment). Many mums find that expressing after a feed works best. This milk can either be chilled in the fridge for up to 48 hours or frozen for up to three months for later use.

Pumps can be bought at the pharmacy, and some breast-feeding organisations lend out pumps, usually for a small charge, as electric pumps are expensive.

There are many pumps on the market but the important thing to remember is that they must be sterilised before each use and you will need to follow the instructions for correct assembly and usage. This is a job your partner could take responsibility for, as the pump needs to be 'built' before each use, and it is much better to be handed the pump sterilised, assembled and ready to go. Even if you prefer to express whilst your partner is at work, they could always get it ready for you before they go in the morning.

Leaking milk

Leaking varies enormously for many women: some mums find a crying baby (not always their own) causes leaking and can't leave the house without breast pads; other women have only a little leak now and then. Most women do need to use breast pads inserted in their bra to cope with leaking between feeds in the first months of breastfeeding, as this is when milk production is highest.

When there have been some hours between feeds, leaking is often copious and the first feed of the morning may soak your clothes whilst you are feeding from the first side, so it can be helpful to insert a muslin (soft cotton) cloth into your nightdress or top to mop up the milk if you haven't had the chance to put on your bra and a breast pad yet.

A little consolation for all this dampness is that you are producing lots of milk for your baby. You'll find that when weaning starts and you start to reduce the number of times you feed a day you'll leak less and may not need to wear breast pads any more.

Colic

You will be able to see if it is colic that is making your baby cry when they draw up their knees, arch their back or try to push themselves off your lap or out of your arms with their feet. Keeping a firm hold will keep them safe and secure. To calm them you may want to try the Up-Down Technique (see Chapter 3) to get them to stop crying – dads are usually great at this.

Try soothing your Little One: babies love sympathy. If you calmly tell them Mummy or Daddy is here and you know how hard it is, it will help focus your mind and give them comfort to get over the colic spasm quickly. It is hard for your baby when they have colic, as they don't understand what this pain is, and they don't know it will pass soon enough.

Colic, which literally means 'pain', is horrid for your baby and for you. Your Little One is experiencing the discomfort of digestion for the first time. Just picture all the rumblings in their tummy and the windy feeling as a brand-new gut has to digest all the nutrients from their milk. Their bodies are learning how to do this, and your baby's problem is gas, not you. I know it's horrible when they get beside themselves with colic, but your baby has no idea what is causing this pain and does not know when it will end. It comes as a bit of a shock for them after all those months of a carefree existence in the womb.

You can give your Little One some relief by staying calm and giving them lots of comfort; it may be you want to try some skin-to-skin contact so they can feel your warmth and hear your heartbeat.

There are products on the market to help relieve colic, and your doctor or health visitor can write you a prescription or you can get over-the-counter remedies from the pharmacist.

There are remedies you give to your baby before the feed which work by bringing all the little bubbles of wind together to help your baby to burp them up, and they may posset and vomit up a little milk as well which is to be expected with these products.

You can also use gripe water from the ages of six to eight weeks by giving a 2.5 ml spoon in 1 fl oz of cooled boiled water in a sterilised bottle. I usually say gripe water works best when your Little One is experiencing colic as it will help to bring up any wind if you give it to them 10–15 minutes before their feed, and make it more likely they'll have an easier job finishing their milk.

What works for your baby may not be the same as for your friends' babies, so keep an open mind and use only one product at a time. I have known mums who have been having such a hard time and are so desperate to find a remedy they've given all the products together, but not only would this mean you wouldn't know which product worked for your baby, it would be unsafe as well. (See the A–Z section for further information.)

Posseting

Posseting is common in most babies and is an old-fashioned word that we use for babies who bring up little bits of vomit after feeding or sometimes even during a feed. It is normal for babies to posset because, as they burp, often some partly digested feed comes up. Many babies will be experiencing symptoms of colic as well as posseting from birth to six months, so it is no wonder it makes many parents feel anxious. Posseting is nothing to worry about unless you think it is affecting your baby's weight gain and well-being.

You cannot stop your baby being sick but you can help them by feeding frequently (usually every two to three hours); raising the head end of their crib by placing a folded blanket or muslin underneath their mattress so your baby can rest in a more upright position; and giving your baby the opportunity to be on their tummy during regular supervised 'Tummy Time'. Once they can sit up with support, being upright may help lessen their vomiting reflex. Once babies start to wean and are having solid food and spend more of their day in an upright position, most parents notice they posset less or not at all.

Reflux

A small number of babies have Gastro-Oesophageal Reflux Disease (GORD) when acid from the stomach leaks out and backs up into the oesophagus. Sometimes this is confused with posseting, which is very common in new babies who frequently posset or vomit up some of their milk feed during or after a feed. In babies, reflux occurs when the milk feed 'flows back' up the baby's food pipe and is either projectile-vomited or, in the case of silent reflux, is regurgitated back up in the oesophagus and swallowed again.

Reflux requires a professional medical diagnosis and treatment as the acid reflux may cause inflammation of your baby's food pipe and affect their weight gain. If you think your baby has reflux and are worried they are not gaining weight and are in pain and distress, ask for a referral to a paediatrician to investigate and treat if needed.

Tongue-tie

Tongue-tie is when the *frenulum*, a short string-like membrane under the tongue, is tightly attached to the floor of the mouth rather than loosely attached. If your baby has trouble sticking out their tongue and it doesn't go past their gums, or pulls into a heart shape, they may be tongue-tied. If your baby latches on and feeds well, and is gaining weight, they may not need any treatment. However, if your baby finds latching difficult and is not feeding well, ask your health visitor or doctor about whether they think it would help to clip the frenulum.

Winding

Wind is a build-up of gases in the stomach. With all the feeding your baby does there is inevitably a lot of wind in their tummy which causes gripe pains. By winding and burping your baby you are helping them to bring up some of that gas so they feel more relaxed and happier. (Winding techniques are described in the A–Z section.)

Moving on from breastfeeding when the time is right for you

There is no perfect time to give up breastfeeding; it is simply when the time is right for you. Many mums will experience a moment that signifies breastfeeding is coming to an end. It may be for practical reasons like returning to work, or it may be when biting becomes a problem, or that weaning is so established your baby is not showing much interest in breast milk these days. Don't worry about what your friends are doing; some women may only breastfeed for the first few weeks; others will go on until their child is one or over. Whatever you decide, your baby has benefited hugely from the nourishment and time you have given them.

How to manage giving up breastfeeding if your baby is 0–6 months

If in the early weeks of breastfeeding you feel you want to stop and completely switch to formula, do try and drop one feed at a time if you can, rather than suddenly stopping altogether, which makes it hard on you physically (you'll experience engorgement) and your baby (who will need time to adjust to taking formula from a bottle).

You may want your partner or someone else to give the bottle to start with, as it can be confusing for your baby to smell the milk on you and taste the formula at the same time. Once they are used to it, most babies will happily take the bottle of formula from Mum and some won't care who gives it to them just so long as they get their milk. Do whatever is right for you and your baby. (You'll find some helpful advice on bottle feeding in the next chapter.)

Strategies for giving up breastfeeding if your baby is over 6 months old

For mums who want to switch to formula from six months, it is best to drop one feed at a time and replace with a bottle. Babies who are weaning still need regular milk feeds, but when you give them is trial and error. Often it is the middle feed of the day that is easiest to switch first of all from breast to bottle. Your Little One should be easily taking their bottle before you drop another breastfeed. When you are both ready, try replacing the mid-morning breastfeed with a bottle, and then the mid-afternoon or tea-time feed. Pick the feeds where it makes sense or feels right to give the bottle. I know mums who've dropped the tea-time feed first because that is when their partner gets home from work and they can give the bottle instead.

The last feeds to go are usually the early-morning feed and finally the last feed before bed.

How long you take to do this is up to you. It may be that for practical reasons such as returning to work it is something that has to be done over a few weeks. Alternatively, you may have the time to make a gradual change over months.

Dropping the breastfeeds one at a time sounds easy but it can be an emotional and challenging time for many women. You may have your own feeling of loss and even grief when switching to the bottle even if you have been expressing milk, or it might be a huge relief – there is no right or wrong way to feel. Giving up breastfeeding is a decision only you can make. Don't put too much pressure on yourself and, if you can, go with the flow (no pun intended!). Look at the positives – you may find you have more energy, less of an appetite, or just a bit more time to yourself. Trust yourself; you love your baby more than anyone, so have confidence in your own skills and intuitive feelings, and you and your baby will settle into this new method and way of feeding. (For further advice on formula feeding or when to switch to cows' milk, take a look at the next chapter.)

Trust Yourself Checklist

Here's a few reminders for you to check off, so you can trust that you are doing everything you can to successfully breastfeed your baby.

❑ Positioning – is the position you are using ensuring your baby is properly latched on and feeding for as long as they need?

❑ Patience – are you setting aside time to feed where you feel comfortable and relaxed to help reduce frustration and anxiety?

❑ Perseverance – are you taking it a day at a time, recognising the achievement of each day's breastfeeding?

❑ Are you aware of the three signs that your baby is getting enough milk?

2

The Secrets for Successful Bottle-feeding

Both formula- and breastfeeding mums can use bottles to feed their baby. Whether you choose to bottle-feed from the start, after a few weeks, months or at an age when your baby can go straight onto cows' milk, I know you'll want to do the best for your baby. One of the most common issues mums who are bottle-feeding have told me they experience is feeling judged – that people think they are a bad mum because they aren't breastfeeding their baby. Your decision to formula-feed is your business and no one else's; you don't need to explain yourself to other people (it doesn't matter whether you are formula-feeding because you had difficulties breastfeeding or if it was something you didn't feel was right for you – you don't have to justify yourself to other people whether they are friends, family or even health professionals!).

Once you've started to bottle-feed, for whatever reason, embrace it and just look at all the positive things you are doing for your Little One every day. It may help if you let the people supporting you know if you feel guilty or that you are being judged. They will more than likely tell you what a good mum you are, and help create a shield from unwelcome comments.

Bonding with your baby during bottle-feeds

I know some mums do worry that if they aren't breast-feeding they won't be able to bond with their baby, but when you feed your baby with their bottle this can be a wonderful opportunity to connect and enjoy each other. Making the most of this one-on-one time will really make a difference.

Look into your baby's eyes, hold their gaze, sing to them, talk to them and hold their tiny hand. Your baby knows your voice so well; they heard it while they were in your womb, and will get a lot of reassurance from just being close to you, hearing your heartbeat and the sound of your breathing. This will help to encourage attachment between you and your baby, and dads can get in on the act, too.

Bottle-feeding in a calm and relaxed environment where you and your baby can focus on each other will have huge benefits. Enjoy this time, and the extra cuddles you can give them while winding them as you rub their back – it is all precious time between you and your baby. You'll find a feeding technique and a space that is right for you. There is no reason why you can't use feeding time to put your feet up and enjoy some quality time together.

Working with your partner as a team

If your partner does want to do their share of bottle-feeds, that is great news. It'll give you a break and help them establish a stronger connection with the baby. I have known dads who've held back because they are worried they'll break the baby. OK, you do need to be gentle, and I know dropping your baby is sometimes a big fear, but as long as you are sensible all will be well. Babies are very resilient so don't be afraid to handle your Little One – you both will be experts in no time, and they will love a bit of daddy time.

Be gentle, but hold your baby securely. Often dads have a deft touch when it comes to comforting the baby; this may be because the hold is firmer.

Trust Yourself

Enjoy Feeding Time

Feeding time is the perfect time for babies to bond with their parents. Give yourself a bit of time to put your feet up, put some relaxing music on, dim the lights and take some time out with your baby.

Parenthood is a partnership; you could take it in turns to feed and then swap over to settle – just do whatever works for you.

If you are still producing a little breast milk it is often best if your partner gives the baby their formula milk and settles them. The smell of the breast milk may cause your baby to search for it and become confused, and this makes it harder for mums to feed and comfort their Little One. So working together when possible at feeding time will give your Little One more opportunity to adapt and get the milk they need.

If you've stopped breastfeeding it may take several days to completely stop producing milk, so stopping suddenly is not the best way. Try to replace one breastfeed at a time with a bottle, and then drop another every few days so you can have switched over in about one to two weeks.

If you feel that your breasts are hard and engorged, talk to your doctor to see if you need any medication to help.

Getting the right equipment for bottle-feeding

Whenever you choose to start giving your baby a bottle you are going to need a few things to get bottle-feeding underway.

Bottle-feeding Shopping List

The right size teats (sizes 1–3)
Bottles
Steriliser
Muslin
Bottle brush
Washing-up liquid
Pair of Marigolds

Washing up and sterilising safely

As well as bottles, teats and the formula milk, you'll need a steriliser and a bottle brush for washing that is never used for general washing up.

1 Always wash the bottles and teats thoroughly as it is not possible to sterilise something that is not clean first.

2 Wash in warm soapy water very thoroughly.

3 Rinse in cold water afterwards to remove soap residue.

Then always follow the manufacturer's instructions to sterilise.

Choosing the right size teat for a bottle

Your baby needs to have a teat which gives them their milk efficiently; if it is too slow it can cause wind and slow down their feeding, or if it is too fast they can cough and splutter a little bit. Each size increases the flow of the milk, so the older your baby gets the faster they'll be able to down that milk. You'll get a sense of how long your Little One will take to have their feed.

How to make up a bottle of formula

There are several formulas on the market and the choice is yours as to which one you use. What goes into formula milk is adapted as time goes on, so if your mum tells you she always fed you on brand X, it won't be the same formula it was then, so use whatever you want, it's just a question of choice.

How much formula should I use?

The thing with formula milk is that the instructions on the packet are only a guide. Your baby will have their own requirements, so it's important to discuss how to make up the bottles and the amount they need with your midwife or health visitor. If your baby is past the newborn stage, whether you are new to formula-feeding or just want to be sure your

Making Up a Bottle of Formula

1. Use water that has been freshly drawn, boiled and cooled (although the water does still need to be hot emough to dissolve the powder).

2. Always put the water in first and count the number of scoops you use.

3. Add in the same number of scoops of formula as water, e.g. 3 fl oz (90 ml) of water to 3 level scoops of formula, or 4 fl oz (120 ml) of water to 4 level scoops is just right.

4. Put the top on the bottle and shake. Cool it down rapidly as it will be too hot to give to your baby straight away.

5. Test the temperature on the inner part of your arm to feel how warm it is before you give the bottle to your baby, and be careful it's not too hot.

Little One is getting all they need, don't hold back – talk to a health professional (it's what they're there for!).

Never be tempted to put in an extra scoop of formula powder, as it over-concentrates the salts and nutrients and can lead to hypernatremia* very quickly.

Babies can have cold formula as well if needs be. There is also ready-made formula available but this is more expensive than making it up yourself, so just do whatever is right for you at the time.

* Hypernatremia is an elevated sodium (salt) level in the blood.

Perfecting your bottle-feeding technique

Always ensure that all the formula feed is at the top end the bottle with no gaps for air to get in for the perfect bottle-feeding position. Before you start a feed, check you have everything

that you will need at arm's length. Using feeding time to have a much-needed sit-down gives you more time to bond with your baby; so get comfy with a cushion for back support and a footstool if you want one. Fewer demands on you during feeding time will also give you the opportunity to tune in to how your baby feeds and whether you need to make any little adjustments. After feeding, your baby may need winding (winding techniques are in the A–Z section).

Your baby may take the bottle with no hesitation and suck away merrily, but some babies do not open their mouths easily and can be challenging to feed. If your baby seems to be angry or upset and cries and refuses to take the teat, put the bottle aside. Settle them using the Up-Down Technique (in Chapter 3) and wait till you're both calm to try again.

How many feeds does my baby need?

It'll take a little bit of trial and error, and timings and quantities will change as they grow, but if you work towards getting these things in place you'll be well ahead of the game. Having a timetable in your head to help you shape your day is helpful, but babies sometimes don't fit the mould of a strict feeding schedule, though you'll notice patterns emerging. Here's what you can do to get off to a flying start with formula-feeding.

Frequency of feeds

Do feed your baby on demand, but be careful not to let your baby go more than four hours in the daytime without a feed. As you can imagine, your baby's stomach is only as big as their tiny clenched fist, so roughly, depending on the baby's weight, try 2–3 oz (60–90 ml) every two to three hours at first, and then 3–4 oz (90–120 ml) every three to four hours when you feel they can go a bit longer between feeds.

The quantities and frequency of feeding change all the time, and no doubt you'll find that your Little One's needs do vary. If you use a timeframe of no more than four hours between feeds during the daytime in the early weeks, it may help you to avoid having to do frequent feeding at night. Sometimes, especially if a baby is jaundiced, they may be sleepy and will sleep longer than three to four hours. Once they have reached four hours since the start of the last feed, just pop their legs out of their babygro and take off their blanket to let the cool air wake them up naturally. If they are being a real sleepyhead, talk to your Little One and gently move them to wake them up to feed. (Make sure you've made

Trust Yourself

Has Your LO Had Enough?

Babies feed on demand and have an inner clock that tells them when to feed and how much to have. Listen to your baby – they'll tell you when they are hungry and when they are full.

I remember when ... I was a student health visitor nearing the end of my training. We could choose another part of the UK to work in for two weeks of alternative practice and I requested South Wales. I stayed with my sister Bridget in the Gower and was fortunate enough to be assigned to a very experienced health visitor in the Mumbles. It was very different to where I had been working, as 95 per cent of mums in the community regularly attended baby clinic after the primary visit, and generally you didn't visit them at home unless there was a serious problem because home visits provoked a certain amount of curtain-twitching from the neighbours. At one baby clinic a mum arrived with a three-month-old baby. He was a very good size and his mother said to the health visitor, 'I've just started to put a teaspoon of sugar in every feed; that's not wrong, is it?' I was shocked and full of youthful verve, and would have told her it was completely wrong, and what did she think she was doing? But my teacher knew better; she gave a wry smile and said, 'Well, it's not wrong, but these new formulas have everything a baby could need, so you don't need to trouble yourself to put the sugar in any more.' I realised that she had the wisdom to create a win/win solution for mother and baby. Rather than scolding the mother and making her feel embarrassed, she used diplomacy to help the woman save face and ensure the baby wasn't being given sugar with his formula. All the mothers I have met in recent years have been very careful about making up the formula, and often tell me they have to ignore the advice of their grannies who tell them to 'put a rusk in every bottle'. I often think back to all the lovely mums I met in Wales, who were really dedicated to their babies.

up a bottle ready to go – they won't want to wait once they've been woken up!)

The timing of feeds affects your baby's sleep

This shift in when your baby wants to feed may not happen instantly, and sometimes a baby will go down to sleep at, say, 8 pm, and sleep through for a short time, but may then suddenly be awake several times a night. Parents often don't associate this with the timing of feeds, but the two are often related. Patience and perseverance are what's needed from you and your partner to get your baby sleeping and feeding well.

Solutions to common bottle-feeding problems

Taking too long to feed or not finishing their bottle

If you find your baby is taking longer and longer to feed from the bottle and is labouring over it more and more, this may be because the teat flow is too slow. It may be time to switch to a number 2 or 3 size teat or variflow-type teat to help your Little One get their milk at the speed that is right for them.

On average it takes a baby 15–20 minutes to drink a bottle of milk and they shouldn't really be taking longer than 30–35 minutes, because the baby will most likely become tired and frustrated and even give up, which would mean they wouldn't be getting all the milk they need.

When a baby takes a long time to feed it can also cause wind, which gets them annoyed and makes the whole process a lot harder. So if your baby is taking too long, switch the teat first and, if problems persist, you might want to try changing the brand of formula you are using.

Colic

The movement of the teeth through your baby's jaw and gums as the early teething pains kick in often happens at the same time as they experience colic. With all this going on, babies need massive amounts of reassurance and comforting. You will be able to see if it is colic that is making your baby cry by signs such as if they draw up their knees, arch their back or try to push themselves off your lap or out of your arms with their feet. Keeping a firm hold will keep them safe and secure. To calm them you may want to try the Up-Down Technique (see Chapter 3) to get them to stop crying – dads are usually great at this.

Try soothing your Little One: babies love sympathy. If you calmly tell them Mummy or Daddy is here and you know how hard it is, it will help focus your mind and give them comfort to get over the colic spasm quickly. It is hard for your baby when they have colic, as they don't under-stand what this pain is, and they don't know it will pass soon enough.

Colic is horrid for your baby and for you. Your Little One is experiencing the discomfort of digestion for the first time. Just picture all the rumblings in their tummy and the windy feeling as a brand-new gut has to digest all the nutrients from their milk. Their bodies are learning how to do this, and your baby's problem is gas, not you. I know it's horrible when they get beside themselves with colic, but your baby has no idea what is causing this pain and does not know when it will end.

It comes as a bit of a shock for them after all those months of a carefree existence in the womb.

You can give them some relief by staying calm and giving them lots of comfort; it may be you want to try some skin-to-skin contact so they can feel your warmth and hear your heartbeat.

There are products on the market to help relieve colic, and your doctor or health visitor can write you a prescription or you can get over-the-counter remedies from the pharmacist.

You can choose products that go into the formula to break down the curds, as it were, or remedies that you give to your baby before the feed which work by bringing all the little bubbles of wind together to help your baby to burp them up, and they may posset and vomit up a little milk as well, which is to be expected with these products.

You can also use gripe water from the ages of six to eight weeks by giving a 2.5 ml spoon in 1 fl oz of cooled boiled water in a sterilised bottle. I usually say gripe water works best when your Little One is experiencing colic as it will help to bring up any wind if you give it to them 10–15 minutes before their formula feed, and make it more likely they'll have an easier job finishing their bottle of milk.

What works for your baby may not be the same as for your friends' babies, so keep an open mind and use only one product at a time. I have known mums who been having such a hard time and are so desperate to find a remedy they've given all the products together, but not only would this mean you wouldn't know which product worked for your baby, it would be unsafe as well.

Posseting

Posseting is common in most babies and is an old-fashioned word that we use for babies who bring up little bits of vomit after feeding or sometimes even during a feed. It is normal for babies to posset because, as they burp, often some partly digested feed comes up. Many babies will be experiencing symptoms of colic as well as posseting from birth to six months, so it is no wonder it makes many parents feel anxious. Posseting is nothing to worry about unless you think it is affecting your baby's weight gain and well-being.

You cannot stop your baby being sick but you can help them by feeding frequently (usually every two to three hours); raising the head end of their crib by placing a folded blanket or muslin underneath their mattress so your baby can rest in a more upright position; and giving your baby the opportunity to be on their tummy during regular supervised 'Tummy Time'. Once they can sit up with support, being upright may help lessen their vomiting reflex. Once babies start to wean and are having solid food and spend more of their day in an upright position, most parents notice they posset less or not at all.

Reflux

A small number of babies have Gastro-Oesophageal Reflux Disease (GORD) when acid from the stomach leaks out and back up into the oesophagus. Sometimes this is confused with posseting, which is very common in new babies who frequently posset or vomit up some of their milk feed during or after a feed. In babies, reflux occurs when the milk feed 'flows back' up the baby's food pipe and is either projectile-vomited or, in the case of silent reflux, is regurgitated back up in the oesophagus and swallowed again.

Reflux requires a professional medical diagnosis and treatment as the acid reflux may cause inflammation of your baby's food pipe and affect their weight gain. If you think your baby has reflux and are worried they are not gaining weight and are in pain and distress, ask for a referral to a paediatrician to investigate and treat if needed.

Tongue-tie

Tongue-tie is when the *frenulum*, a short string-like membrane under the tongue, is tightly attached to the floor of the mouth rather than loosely attached. If your baby has trouble sticking out their tongue and it doesn't go past their gums, or pulls into a heart shape, they may be tongue-tied. If your baby latches on and feeds well, and is gaining weight, they may not need any treatment. However, if your baby is not feeding well, ask your health visitor or doctor about whether they think it would help to clip the frenulum.

Winding

Wind is a build-up of gases in the stomach. With all the feeding your baby does there is inevitably a lot of wind in their tummy which causes gripe pains. By winding and burping your baby you are helping them to bring up some of that gas so they feel more relaxed and happier. (Winding techniques are described in the A–Z section.)

Moving from a bottle to a beaker or cup

When your baby begins to wean it is worth trying a baby beaker. Put a little cooled boiled water into a very clean sippy or tippy cup when you feel the time is right, just to get them familiar with holding it and to have a bit of fun at drinking on their own. It's great to give babies new experiences, and this is new to them.

Some babies take to drinking from a beaker or a cup straight away, while others won't even entertain it. Offer them the beaker, and don't worry if they don't want to take it; they will when they are ready. Just placing it on their high-chair tray or giving them it to hold whilst you are getting their lunch ready is opportunity enough (you'll want something with a lid to start with!).

If your baby doesn't like it, just leave it for a week before you try again, and try, try, try again once a week to give them the opportunity without expectations or pressure. It may be your baby prefers just a little amount in an open plastic beaker with no top, which is great – just have the kitchen roll on hand to mop up the mess. Only give your Little One water; you don't need to give them juice, and if you don't, you'll be doing them a real favour, as the sweet taste of juice lasts for life, and they can wait a bit longer before developing a sweet tooth.

Trust Yourself Checklist

A few reminders so you can trust yourself that bottle-feeding is going well.

❑ Mums and dads can use bottle-feeding for a little one-on-one time. Using this time to bond with your baby willl pave the way for attachment as your baby develops during their first year.

❑ We all know mums can do three things at once, but using feeding time to relax and connect with your baby and focus on them is a real opportunity for you both to have a little R&R time.

❑ Take the bottle apart, wash it throughly so it is squeaky clean and then pop it in the steriliser. This is the only way to ensure bottle-feeding equipment is sterilised.

❑ Take a little time now and again to consider if you are using the right size teat for your baby by considering how often and for how long they are feeding.

❑ Follow the formula instructions and always check the temperature before giving your baby a bottle.

3

Sleep, Calming and Creating Your Own Routine

All babies vary in the amount of sleep they need and their sleeping patterns. You'll find different techniques work for different times of the day or depending on where you are (a nice quiet shady nursery is a very different place from a noisy and busy bus or café when it's time for the Sandman to come). Mums and dads will often have slightly different methods of getting the baby off to sleep, and having a variety of techniques up your sleeve certainly comes in handy. As your Little One grows and changes, so will their preference for how they like to fall asleep; when they are newborn it is often only a feed and a cuddle that will get them off, but as they get older a story and some soothing music may be more likely to do the trick.

It's important to use the calming and sleep techniques you feel comfortable with; what works for you as a family might not work for other people and vice versa. As with most things there is no one right way to get your baby off to sleep – it's about choice and your circumstances in the moment. Some days are easier than others and I know it can be especially hard when you are desperate for a little shut-eye yourself. We'll look at some tried-and-tested methods I've come across for getting a baby to stop crying or into the land of nod. Just do the ones you want to have a go at; some will work for your Little One and others won't ... every baby is different ... and with a little patience and perseverance you'll find the right way for you and your baby.

All babies cry

It is normal for babies to cry and part and parcel of parenthood, but there's crying and there's non-stop wailing which means your Little One is in distress about something. An assessment of what is causing your baby to cry followed by swift action will often mean those tears will be short lived. A cuddle, a calm and soothing voice, and a bit of sympathy will usually help you both relax.

During the first few months babies will often cry if they are hungry or suffering from colic, wind or teething pain (you will find remedies for these in the A–Z). Later on your Little One may cry if you leave the room, as part of their developing feelings of attachment and their need to have you close by. If you are anxious and do not understand what is making your baby cry, just make a note of the signs and symptoms you are seeing and call your health visitor, doctor or midwife. It may lead to an appointment to check the baby if that's needed, or they may tell you everything is normal and to be expected. It's fine to ask questions and raise any concerns, as there are hundreds of things that parents see and ask themselves, 'Is this normal?' and in a lot of cases the answer is, 'Yes,' but it is your right to ask your health professional, so go ahead. Sometimes solutions for your concerns are only a phone call away. Never worry that they will think you are wasting their time, as they most probably can identify any problems and reassure you that all is well.

Do trust your own judgement and intuition about your baby, ask questions and raise any concerns you have. Parents know their baby best, so you will get to know what is wrong when they are upset and crying, and be more than capable of using your intuition to try ways to settle and soothe your Little One. Try not to be self-critical and think you are a bad parent – all babies cry.

Tips for calming a crying baby

Whether it's time to go to bed or your baby is crying for a feed and you need just a few more minutes to get everything ready, here are a few tips you can try to take the pressure off, as no one likes to hear their baby cry, no matter how short lived it may be. Many of these techniques can be combined to comfort yourself and your baby. Your Little One won't be able to sleep, eat, have a bath or go out for a walk unless they are calm, and that means you need to be calm, too. That's why taking a few deep breaths, lowering your shoulders and reminding yourself that all babies cry before you try and settle your baby will help both of you. Sometimes it means stopping in your tracks and being a bit late, but swift action to soothe and meet your baby's needs means you'll all be happier for it.

My instant calmer for a happy baby

The Up-Down Technique is a forgotten baby-calming trick that recreates the weightlessness and comfort of being in the womb and can stop a baby crying in a couple of minutes or even a few seconds. Dads are often the best person to put this technique into practice as it requires some arm power to do for even a few minutes (giving you a mini-workout at home!). It's a good calming technique to use to get your baby to stop crying and then you can start to feed them or get ready to go out.

Stand up. Hold your baby with one hand under their bottom, placing your thumb and forefinger gently round their thigh and resting the baby's head in the palm of your other hand. When your Little One feels secure, move them up and down, slightly away from your body, using a rapid up-and-down motion. You will usually find they'll stop crying in moments. Your baby will probably start crying again when you stop the movement, but may be calm enough to start a feed or, if they are tired, to go to sleep.

Try these calming techniques to comfort and soothe your Little One

There is no one way calm a baby. Trust your instincts and do what feels right. Most parents instinctively combine these techniques to calm and reassure their baby.

Take a deep breath and sway

Holding your baby against your chest with their head on your shoulder, gently sway and take a deep breath, filling your chest so the air pushes out your stomach, and then exhale, pushing all the air out and drawing your abdomen in. Repeat at least ten times, dropping your shoulders down and away from your ears and closing your eyes if you want to. As your body begins to relax, so will your baby.

Talking it through

When your baby is distressed you can calm you both down by gently talking to them and giving them lots of sympathy. Soothe them by describing what's happening; telling them it

Happy Baby Up-Down Technique

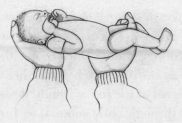

1 Gently rest baby's head in the palm of your hand and hold their bottom in the palm of the other hand, wrapping thumb and forefinger around the baby's thigh.

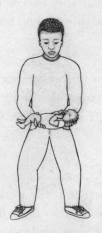

2 Stand with your feet hip-width apart with the baby at waist height.

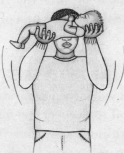

3 Move baby up to shoulder height and back down again to waist height in a rapid motion and repeat for a couple of minutes.

will be over soon and you're here for them and love them will all serve as a gentle reminder and distraction for both of you.

Lay them on your chest

In the daytime when you are not in danger of falling asleep yourself, your baby will always prefer to rest on you and to listen to your heartbeat and breathing. Many babies favour the left side when lying on your chest, as the sound of your heart beating is soothing and reminiscent of life in the womb. Resist the urge to always settle them through body contact, as further on parents can find it is the only way they can calm and get their baby to sleep and you can't use this method forever.

Skin to skin

You can always go back to skin to skin to soothe your baby. The warmth and closeness is a lovely reminder of the bond you share and can be really comforting for your Little One in times of distress.

Music

Singing a lullaby or playing gentle music can really work wonders on some babies. You'll soon learn what your baby likes to hear, and if you sang and played music a lot while they were in the womb it's quite likely they'll like those tunes best of all.

Baby massage

It is worth trying a little massage to calm and comfort your baby. Just gently massaging their feet when then are fretting in the crib may send your Little One off to sleep, or you might want to incorporate it into your bathtime or bedtime routine. Use a little neutral baby moisturiser on your hands, not baby oil (classes may use a little massage oil, but at home the moisturiser is just to protect your baby's soft skin). Use the flat of your hands to gently massage your baby; they will enjoy the warm and light pressure of your touch as you gently press their thigh, leg, ankle, foot and each tiny toe, starting with the big one, and it is a lovely way to bond with your Little One. There are often postnatal massage classes if you want to get some instruction and the opportunity to meet other mums; otherwise just use your common sense.

Walk around with them in a sling or baby carrier

Useful in the day, particularly if you need your hands free or have a few errands to run. If you decide to try using the sling it is well worth getting some instruction on how best to use it safely and effectively. There may be a sling meeting in your area, and there are videos online. If you opt for a baby carrier then just follow the instructions and weight guidelines and pop them in (dads are often a big fan of these ... and it does look very cute). If you have any back problems, do take medical advice before use.

Fresh air and travel

Babies who get out in the fresh air on a daily basis have much more chance of sleeping well at night. Even on a rainy day you may want to try taking your baby out in the car as they will often fall asleep. The soothing motion frequently induces slumber when they are in the pram, buggy, car or bus.

Swing chairs

Under constant daytime supervision and for only short periods of time, there are swing chairs that rock a baby, play music and can be a nice calming experience for your baby. Usually they only want to be in for 5 to 10 minutes.

Shush, shush, shush

This is not about telling your baby to pipe down, but making gentle, rhythmic shushing sounds will often help them to relax. It simulates the noises of blood pumping as babies like sounds and sensations that are reminiscent of the womb. From gently behind the ear, not into the ear, make low-level rhythmic shushing noises for a couple of minutes to calm your Little One.

I remember when ... the Australian soap opera *Neighbours* was popular lunchtime and tea-time viewing. Pregnant women would often put their feet up and relax to enjoy the show. I found there was a whole generation of infants who stopped crying when they heard the *Neighbours* theme song as a tune assoicated with relaxation and calm from their days in the womb.

Sleeping and feeding go hand in hand

When babies are new it can feel like life is an endless round of feeding, winding, nappy-changing and crying. Often parents find the sleeping bit isn't happening as much as you'd like, especially at night when you've never needed 40 winks more. Most babies are fed on demand because babies have an inner clock which is set by their own unique needs for feeding. That's why even though it's really helpful to have expectations that your Little One will feed frequently, the exact timing is not going to follow a textbook scenario in the early weeks and months. It usually takes a little trial and error to settle and discover your baby's pattern for feeding, which constantly shifts so you'll often have an ever-evolving routine.

A newborn baby usually feeds every two to three hours and sometimes even more frequently in the first few weeks, depending on their individual needs. Your Little One's tiny stomach is only the size of their clenched fist. Hopefully, as your baby becomes more efficient at feeding they will stretch to feeding every three to four hours.

Getting the right amount of nap time and milk during the day is part of the secret to a good night's sleep. Let your baby have a maximum of four hours between feeds during the day. If they are napping then you can gently encourage them to wake up (so they don't get too much sleep in the day and don't miss a feed). Frequent feeding during the day often means your Little One will wake less frequently in the night. It is normal for a newborn baby to wake to feed in the night because they don't have a concept of night and day, only the inner clock that demands feeding.

Trust Yourself

Waking a Sleepy Baby during the Day

If your baby is due a feed you can encourage them to wake naturally by popping their legs out of their clothing and removing any blankets so they can feel the cool air on their little feet and legs. Talking softly to your baby and turning the light up a bit will encourage them to wake gently and gradually so they can get their feed. So, do feed on demand but try to ensure that in the daytime there is never longer than a four-hour gap between feeds.

Your baby's cry is their way of telling you something is wrong

Though it is important to recognise that all babies cry, there is a difference between grumping off to sleep and a cry of distress. Leaving your baby to grump off to sleep for about five minutes or so is fine, but if they aren't asleep after 15 minutes and are wailing for you, I would not advocate leaving a baby to cry themselves to sleep. If they are feeling insecure, or are in pain, or hungry, then leaving them to cry all night is not going to make for a happy, well-attached baby in the long term. Some parents will tell you they left their baby to cry for a few nights and they soon learned to go through, and for me that's the crux of it – 'they *learned* not to cry'. To develop a lifelong bond with your child that is positive, well-balanced and nurturing, they need to learn that you are there for them. (You can read more about why your baby needs your attention and about the long-term benefits of meeting your child's emotional needs in Chapter 6.)

Safe sleep

Even though it's nice to be warm and cosy, it's important that babies don't get too hot as they can't regulate their own body temperature until they are at least 18 months to two years old. You need to be within earshot of your Little One while they sleep. If they aren't in the room with you, always use a baby monitor.

Making up their bed

Whether they are in a crib or a pram, babies should always sleep on their backs with their feet touching the bottom end of the cot, so their toes touch the end. Covers should be no higher than your Little One's shoulders, and tuck them in securely so the covers can't slip over their head. Never use a duvet, quilt or pillow for a baby, and in very hot weather your baby may only need a sheet. I prefer making up their bed with only blankets and sheets, but the choice of the bedding you want to use is yours.

Controlling your baby's temperature

Keeping the room where your baby sleeps at 18°C (65°F) is the recommended temperature. Prevent your baby from over-heating by selecting their clothes and bedding according to how you feel: if you're too hot or too cold, your baby probably is, too. Using layers of lightweight blankets means you can easily adjust your Little One's temperature by adding another layer or taking one away. Babies lose excess heat through their heads, which is why they don't need a hat on when they sleep, even on cold nights. If their body temperature is normal but their hands and feet feel cool, don't worry, this is common. Use how hot or cold their tummy feels as a guide to judging their body temperature. Ensure they never sleep next to a radiator, heater or fire, and never use a hot-water bottle or electric blanket.

Moving your baby into a cot

Babies usually move from a crib to a full-size cot when they have outgrown their Moses Basket or are starting to roll over. You can build up to making the transition by starting to put the basket inside the cot during the day when they are napping so they become familiar with the cot – and their nursery if you are working up to putting your Little One into their own room as well. The same safe sleep rules apply and you should always put your baby down to sleep in their cot on their back with their feet touching the end, tucking in blankets and sheets up to shoulder height. No duvet or pillows are needed.

Ways to help your baby drift off to sleep

The Happy Baby Half Swaddle

Many babies comfort themselves by putting their fingers and thumbs in their mouths and stroking their own face. Using the half swaddle lets your Little One keep their hands free whilst still giving them the secure feeling of being wrapped. Swaddling minimises the thrashing babies do to help them to be stiller and drift off to sleep.

If your baby doesn't object to being wrapped, then swaddling can really help newborn babies feel secure and snug. Most babies like to keep their hands out of the wrap; even if they scratch themselves a bit they will soon learn not to do this any more. Keeping their nails clipped with blunt rounded baby nail scissors helps to prevent this (see the A–Z for more on this).

Spread a large muslin square on a flat surface and lay the baby down with the top of the cloth just under their armpits. Wrap it around them like a bath towel and tuck the end up to keep their feet in and their toes cosy, so they can't kick

Happy Baby Half Swaddle

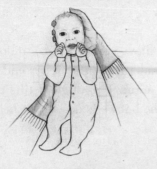

1 Lie the baby on their back on a flat surface with their head over the top edge over a large square cotton muslin.

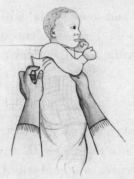

2 Fold one side over and tuck in behind the baby's back so the top edge of the swaddle is under the armpit, leaving both hands free.

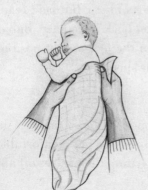

3 Fold across the other side and tuck in at the back. You can fold up the bottom piece and tuck in like an envelope or leave the baby free to kick.

themselves awake or wake up from cold feet. The choice of whether to swaddle or not and how to do it is up to you. I prefer doing the half swaddle as it isn't too restrictive.

Tilt their mattress

Though you should never use a pillow, you can put a pillow, folded sheet, blanket or muslin underneath the upper end of the mattress on their crib, cot or pram. This slightly tilts the mattress and raises the level of the baby's head, which helps their breathing.

Darken the room

If your baby has been fed, changed and soothed and still will not settle, remember to keep the room darkish to encourage and enable sleep to happen by turning the lights down low and drawing the curtains.

Tuck them in

Just check your baby is securely tucked in and that their feet are covered, with the blanket coming no higher than their shoulders to keep your Little One secure, snug and still. If the blanket comes off and your baby starts to stir but isn't ready to wake up, gently re-tuck the blanket back into place. Babies should always sleep on their backs in the feet-to-foot position with the blanket no higher than their shoulders.

Grumping

Not many of us fall asleep the second our head touches the pillow; most of us will take a few minutes to get comfortable. Giving your baby 5 to 10 minutes to grump themselves off and settle down will do them no harm.

Stroke the bridge of their nose

Take your index finger and softly stroke it from your baby's forehead to the middle of their nose. This motion will encourage their eyes to close.

Stroking their forehead and temple or back of the head

Some babies like gentle stroking to their head. This rhythmic motion and the warmth of your touch can be very soothing and help them get off to sleep.

Place a hand on their tummy

If it is night-time and you need your sleep as well, as a last resort place a hand on their tummy if the crib is next to the bed so they have your touch and know you're there.

Rocking chair

Cuddling up with your baby in a rocking chair is one of the most tried-and-tested methods of getting them off to sleep. The combination of your warmth, touch, breathing and heartbeat combined with the gentle rocking motion is a match made in baby heaven.

Rock-a-bye-baby

You can gently rock some Moses Baskets and cribs on a rocking stand. Place your baby in once they are sleepy and calm, and think about combining this with either music, a lullaby, stroking or lightly touching and soothing your baby to sleep.

Put the hoover or hairdryer on

Some babies can drift off rather quickly to the sounds of the hoover or hairdryer. It blocks out other distracting sounds and gives them a mono sound to focus on. Many parents have CDs or apps with white noise, hoover, hairdryer and heartbeat sounds.

Putting them down once they are asleep

Transferring your Little One to a cot once they are asleep by lowering them down slowly and gently whilst you exhale a long breath will keep you relaxed and steady so they don't wake up on the way down. You can also use a strong sheet or blanket as a sling to transfer the baby into their cot. It is a good habit to put the baby into their crib to sleep most of the time.

Place baby's hands on their chest

If your baby wakes as you put them down to sleep, some babies will be calmed if you gently place both their hands on their chest and hold them in place with your hand on top of theirs to still and calm them for a few minutes as you take long deep breaths in and out.

Getting a bit of shut-eye yourself

It often feels as if you never get the unbroken, deep, refreshing sleep that you want and so need; if you get a chance, take a nap when your baby is sleeping. Just 30–40 minutes can make a big difference.

Adaptable mini-routines you can follow and adjust to suit your baby

Meeting your baby's practical needs is all part of the interconnected care that helps them sleep. A newborn baby may feed very frequently and may or may not sleep between feeds. Finding a routine that works for you in the early days may seem very elusive as your Little One's pattern keeps on changing, making it hard to plan or keep pace with your growing baby. You could adapt the following mini-routines depending on what time your baby wakes up. Do mix it up to suit the things you want to do with your baby and what you need to get done in a day ... every day will be a little different.

These examples are mainly based on a baby who feeds every three hours, but if your baby is small or premature they may need to feed every two hours or sometimes more. It's a good idea to have a cut-off point in your head for when you would need to encourage your baby to feed, and it's good to have a general time-frame to help you manage your day, but do still feed on demand. I've put a few suggestions in for activities, but what you do is up to you – it's the feeding and the sleeping that need to find a pattern.

Every baby is different and you'll find that things are constantly shifting in how and when you feed them and put them down for a nap. There will be patterns, though, and getting a mini-routine that is flexible is often helpful so you can shape and influence the day's activities and assure yourself that your Little One is getting everything they need.

Here are some suggestions for possible routines at different ages. They are just a rough guide to be tweaked around you and your family, so always do what works best for you. The start times and time each mini-routine takes will all vary.

Adaptable Mini-Routine (0–3 Weeks)

6.00am – 7.00am	• First feed (breast milk or formula) • Wind and change nappy • Try and put them down in the crib for a sleep and catch up on an extra 40 winks yourself
9.00am – 11.00am	• Second feed • Wind and change nappy • If baby is still awake clean their eyes, face and hands and get them dressed • Gentle play/Tummy Time/singing • Nap time
12.30am – 1.30pm	• Third feed • Wind and nappy change • Maybe a trip out in the fresh air just for a short walk or little time in the baby swing chair with some chatting and singing

2.30pm – 3.30pm	• Fourth feed • Wind and nappy change • Nap time
5.00pm – 7.30pm	• Fifth feed • Wind and nappy change • Maybe a bath • Chatting, singing and playing with daddy • Short nap
8.00pm – 9.00pm	• Sixth feed • Wind and change nappy
11.00pm –12.00am	• Nappy change • Half swaddle in large muslin (if used) • Last feed • Wind • Put baby in crib to sleep

Adaptable Mini-Routine (4–8 Weeks)

Your Little One may start to go for longer between feeds but will still need those naps during the day in order to sleep well at night. Here's an adaptable mini-routine:

6.00am – 7.00am	• First feed • Wind and nappy change • Pop them back to sleep in their crib
9.00am – 10.00am	• Second feed • Wind and nappy change • Clean eyes, face and hands and dress • Go out for some fresh air • Nap time
12.00pm – 1.00pm	• Third feed • Wind and change nappy • Nap time/play/outing

3.00pm – 4.00pm	• Fourth feed • Wind and nappy change • Nap time
6.00pm – 7.00pm	• Fifth feed • Wind and nappy change • Playtime with daddy • Bath time
9.00pm – 10.00pm	• Sixth feed • Wind and nappy change • Little nap
11.30pm – 12.30am	• Nappy change • Half swaddle in a muslin (if used) • Last feed • Wind • Put baby in crib to sleep

Adaptable Mini-Routine (8–12 Weeks)	
6.00am – 7.00am	• First feed • Wind and change nappy • Little bit of extra sleep
9.00am – 10.30am	• Second feed • Wind and nappy change • Wash and dress • Play/outing/story/singing or a little TV • Nap time
12.00am – 1.00pm	• Third feed • Wind and nappy change • Outing/playtime/Tummy Time • Nap time

3.00pm – 5.00pm	• Fourth feed • Wind and nappy change • Nap • Playtime with daddy • Bath
6.30pm – 7.30pm	• Fifth feed • Wind and change nappy • Little nap
10.30pm – 11.30pm	• Nappy change • Half swaddle in muslin (if used) • Last feed • Wind • Put baby in crib to sleep

Adaptable Mini-Routine (12–20 Weeks)

6.00am – 7.00am	• First feed • Wind and nappy change • Pop them back in crib for a little more sleep
9.00am – 10.00am	• Second feed • Wash and dress • Tummy Time/playtime/outing/group/clinic visit
12.00pm – 1.00pm	• Third feed • Wind and nappy change • Play/outing • Nap

3.00pm – 4.00pm	• Fourth feed • Wind and nappy change
6.00pm – 7.00pm	• Fifth feed • Wind • Bath • Gentle play
9.00pm – 11.00pm	• Nappy change • Half swaddle in large muslin (if used) • Last feed • Wind • Put baby in crib to sleep

Adaptable Mini-Routine (6–9 Months)	
6.00am – 8.00am	• First feed
9.00am	• Breakfast • Second feed • Playtime/outing/baby group
12.00pm – 1.00pm	• Lunch
1.30pm – 2.00pm	• Nap or outing
2.30pm – 3.30pm	• Third feed • Playtime/nap/outing

5.00pm – 7.00pm	• Tea • Bath • Playtime
9.00pm – 10.00pm	• Milky supper, e.g. porridge/ unsugared cereal • Nappy change • Feed • Sleep

Adaptable Mini-Routine (9–12 Months)	
6.00am – 8.00am	• Feed if needed or go straight to breakfast • Breakfast (if they haven't had a feed give them some milk in a beaker)
10.00am – 11.00am	• Mid-morning healthy snack • Milk in a beaker
12.00pm – 2.00pm	• Lunch • Outing/playtime/nap
3.00pm – 4.00pm	• Mid-afternoon healthy snack and milk or water in a beaker • Outing/playtime/nap

5.00pm – 7.00pm	• Tea • Bath • Playtime
8.00pm – 9.00pm	• Milky supper, e.g. porridge/ unsugared cereal and milk • Nappy change • Bedtime story • Sleep

4

Being a New Mum Is Life Changing

Becoming a mum is very physically and emotionally demanding; even everyday tasks like washing yourself, cleaning your teeth and finding the time to go to the toilet can feel like a big effort sometimes. It is really important to look after your own health as well as your baby's. Having enough to eat and drink and getting some rest when you can is far more important than housework, though I know we are all different when it comes to chores. Some new mums feel driven to keep the home in pre-baby order, and if this is you then do whatever feels right; it doesn't help when everyone is telling you to let the dust wait if it's getting to you. It's not that having a baby means you should just not bother keeping your home clean and tidy; of course you want a lovely environment for your baby; but if you can, try and shift some of the responsibility so you can focus on your new baby as it will help take away unnecessary pressure. It might be that your partner or family take on a bit more, or if you can afford it get a cleaner to help for a few weeks. If you can't get any help, try and just do the essentials and leave doing the cupboards for a while.

Relationships between you and your partner, your family and friends all seem to shift when your new baby makes their début and it can be a very emotionally charged time. Many mums and dads feel very protective of their new baby and feel unsure about handing them over to anyone else. Some families want time and privacy to adjust to their new life as a family within their own home, and for the time being outsiders aren't welcome. Other new mums feel an urge to get out into the fresh air and feel hemmed in by the four walls of home. These feelings are usually temporary and how you feel can vary from hour to hour, never mind day to day.

When it comes to your feelings for your baby and your love for them, it can be difficult to put it into words. Loving your baby can make you feel grateful, proud, happy and fearful all at the same time, with lots of other feelings mixed in too. When you are exhausted and lacking sleep, emotions can come swiftly to the surface and make you question why you decided to embark on parenthood, but often just the sight of your lovely baby will remind you why. Before we become parents, many people have fixed ideas on bringing up children, often based on their own childhood experiences. When parenthood becomes a 24/7 reality, we often realise there needs to be some flexibility as we find ourselves in situations we could never have envisaged, and that our unique Little One has their own ideas on how things should be, too. It is your opportunity to consciously decide if you want to be positive parents and to recognise what you are doing and can do to have a happy baby and a happy family.

Nearly all new mums feel anxious

You may be feeling up one minute and very down the next, which is normal and to be expected. These feelings can be in the form of anxieties about your baby, yourself, your partner, or new situations and scenarios. There is almost no new mum who doesn't check their baby's breathing frequently – rest assured, almost everyone does it! Feeling very protective and worrying about what might happen is very normal and understandable. Nature wants you to be alert to possible dangers, and that's why these feelings can be very strong.

You may feel at times that the real you has disappeared and that your life is completely consumed by your baby. This is fine for a short time, but happy babies do need happy mummies, so if you are starting to feel overwhelmed, lost or resentful it is best for everyone to find a way to talk about it and try out solutions to relieve these feelings.

Why Do Little Things Affect Me More Than They Used To?

Have you noticed that you …
• get upset by the news?
• react to loud noises or bright light?
• are tipsy after one tiny drink?

Experiencing highly tuned senses after childbirth is nature's way of keeping us alert to dangers that faced our ancestors, and even in this day and age our bodies still respond to perceived dangers, so allow for this in your feelings and actions.

Many new mums find their senses are raised and that things like reports on tragic events are more distressing than they used to be, especially if they involve babies and children.

Having heightened senses could also mean you are sensitive to noise, bright lights and strong smells – any of these could make you feel uncomfortable.

You may find an alcoholic drink goes straight to your head and you can't drink very much any more – this is nature's way of keeping you alert and ready to attend to your baby (mums and dads need to have their wits about them, but the occasional glass of wine or a spritzer is fine).

A little break is good for everyone

It is natural to want to be with your baby, they need you so much, but it doesn't have to be just you who does their care 24/7. As long as your Little One is with someone they have a good relationship with, like your partner or parents, then everything will be fine.

Don't worry if you are a little forgetful sometimes and appointments and everyday tasks often slip your mind. Your brain is programmed to focus on you and your new baby and everything else is superfluous and sometimes slides by. This is to be expected in many of us, but fear not, it won't last forever – though it can be a cause of irritation and concern, particularly if you've always had a good memory.

Feeling lonely on maternity leave

Many mothers have times when they feel lonely during maternity leave. It can be during night feeds, when your are home by yourself or even at the park – it may seem like all the other mums are friends and know what they are doing, it's just you who feels a bit lost sometimes and doesn't fit in. Some people find it easier to make friends; they can go to new groups and just fit in, but many new parents feel shy and don't understand why they don't seem to enjoy mums and toddlers as much as all the other mothers. It's all about choice: try things out and only do what makes you happy.

If you do feel lonely, this doesn't mean that you're not a good mum or aren't enjoying the time you spend with your Little One. It can be a surprise to feel this way; many parents expect to feel tired, to be changing nappies and up in the night, but wanting some adult company is a common feeling. If you've enjoyed being with your colleagues at work and going out in the evening and on weekends with friends and suddenly your life seems completely unrecognisable and you are working round the clock just to meet your baby's needs – it can be a bit of shock. You might feel guilty if you feel this way and scold yourself, 'Surely I should be far too busy with my lovely baby to feel lonely,' but you can't help the way you feel and it shouldn't be something you have to hide.

The friendships that evolve with other mums who have a baby of a similar age can be a great source of support; texting and social networking can also help you let off steam and have a laugh about the trials and tribulations of motherhood and feel a connection with other people whilst still being there for your baby. It's nice to know we aren't the only ones who forget the baby wipes when they go out, or get caught in a torrential downpour without the rain cover for the pram. Talking about your feelings and processing how different your life has become is really helpful, and it's also nice to find someone who will listen to you talk about all those amazing little things your brilliant baby is doing day by day. It's about being happy, and it is important that you are happy, because your happiness is linked to your baby's.

Gaining a greater insight into our own parents and childhood

As a new parent we often find ourselves questioning and coming to a greater understanding about our own childhood experiences and our relationships with our parents. Some new parents experience newfound appreciation for their parents, especially mums. Many of us never realised before just how much our parents loved us and how much they did for us. For other first-time parents it can confirm feelings that their own upbringing was lacking and that their emotional needs and sometimes physical needs were not fully met. If you or your partner did experience poor attachment or little affection from your parents yourself, or felt insecure and unloved at times, it does not mean you will not be good parents yourselves. The fact that you are taking the time to develop a greater understanding of your own Little One's emotional needs means you are consciously working to be the best parent you can be. It is very unlikely that a poor parent would do this.

A new baby can be an opportunity to heal rifts, and sometimes your parents may have the desire to be more involved this time – it is a second chance for them. But their needs are not what matters here, it is you and your baby that matter, and it is your decision how involved you want grandparents to be. If any external involvement is putting you under pressure and making you feel down or negative about yourself, that is not good for you or your Little One. Some grandparents are a real blessing, and only too willing to make meals, do the hoovering, and know when it's time to go and they are getting in the way ... but not everyone is this lucky. What you and your new family need is love and support. If this isn't happening, and you are experiencing upset and anger over the realisation that your childhood was lacking, don't feel this is a reflection on you in any way. You were a child and had no control over your experiences. It can be really helpful to talk to your partner, a sibling, a friend or someone professional. Just do whatever feels right for you.

Not everyone has overwhelming love for their baby straight away

Loving your baby may take longer for some parents and be immediate for others. There is never just one way to bring up children, so whatever your feelings, they are valid for you. Often without warning, the feelings of love for your baby just kick in. If you feel that something is wrong and you feel disconnected, tell your partner, doctor or health visitor and ask for help. These negative feelings don't just happen in the early weeks of motherhood; for some women they can happen later on, so do make sure you act on them. There are many sources of help and advice, and sometimes just knowing you are not alone and there is support and understanding can help. Don't suffer in silence if this is you; take the first step and tell someone. Almost everyone I know has felt bemused and bewildered and detached at some stage during their baby's first year. For some women it's fleeting and soon forgotten, but for others it is not.

There is no need to urge yourself to feel any particular way, and you may find how you feel depends on a lot of outside influences too. It's easy to feel on top of things when the sun is shining, the house is clean and all you have to do is take your baby to the park and can sit on a bench with a coffee and a sandwich; it's a different story when you get drenched as you drudge round the shops with a grumpy infant in preparation for the hordes of family coming to visit at the weekend, as you hastily try and work out how you are going to fit in cooking a meal, tidying the house and taking care of your baby as well, not to mention getting a shower and smartening yourself up. We all have bad days – that doesn't mean you love your baby any less or you are a bad mum.

Feeling depressed doesn't mean you don't love your baby

I have found that if you ask any mum 'How are you?' then nine times out of ten she'll reply, 'Fine,' because what else can you say?! It doesn't matter who asks the question, and it can be difficult to admit even to those closest to us when we are feeling down or overwhelmed. It is really important that the people supporting you know how you are feeling and that you don't feel judged.

For some women, feeling down or depressed is unrelated to how they feel about their baby. It can be difficult if everyone thinks it is the baby who is making you feel unhappy when it's not that at all. If you feel this way, the first step is to discuss these feelings with someone you feel you can confide in and to speak to a health professional. If you feel very down most of the time, do tell someone, and don't suffer in silence. It might be because you are struggling with feeding, or the baby is crying a lot – whatever it is, saying nothing about it will not make it stop. Your feelings really matter.

The Edinburgh Postnatal Depression Scale

Postnatal depression is often talked about but little understood. It can range from feeling a little down and over-anxious to severe anxiety and depression that requires medical supervision. Your health visitor will usually do a quiz with you called the Edinburgh Postnatal Depression Scale (EPDS). The aim of it is to see if you are having feelings of anxiety or depression and to give you the opportunity to talk about your feelings and get further support if you need it.

I remember when ... I'd given a copy of the Edinburgh Postnatal Depression Scale to a mum at clinic to fill in. When I went to visit her a few days later she handed over a rather crumpled piece of paper. I looked up at her, puzzled, and she told me her husband had thrown it in the bin, but she pulled it out the next morning when he went to work. I asked why, and she told me that in the section where it asked, 'Have you blamed yourself unnecessarily when things went wrong?' she'd written, 'No, I blame him.' We both fell about laughing and ticked, 'I have been able to see the funny side of things.'

The EPDS Questions

You may be asked these questions:

In the past 7 days:

1 I have been able to laugh and see the funny side of things:
- ❑ As much as I always could
- ❑ Not quite so much now
- ❑ Definitely not so much now
- ❑ Not at all

2 I have looked forward with enjoyment to things:
- ❑ As much as I ever did
- ❑ Rather less than I used to
- ❑ Definitely less than I used to
- ❑ Hardly at all

3 I have blamed myself unnecessarily when things went wrong:
- ❑ Yes, most of the time
- ❑ Yes, some of the time
- ❑ Not very often
- ❑ No, never

4 I have been anxious or worried for no good reason:
- ❑ No, not at all
- ❑ Hardly ever
- ❑ Yes, sometimes
- ❑ Yes, very often

5 I have felt scared or panicky for no very good reason:
- ❑ Yes, quite a lot
- ❑ Yes, sometimes

❏ No, not much
❏ No, not at all

6 Things have been getting on top of me:

❏ Yes, most of the time I haven't been able to cope at all
❏ Yes, sometimes I haven't been coping as well as usual
❏ No, most of the time I have coped quite well
❏ No, I have been coping as well as ever

7 I have been so unhappy that I have had difficulty sleeping:

❏ Yes, most of the time
❏ Yes, sometimes
❏ Not very often
❏ No, not at all

8 I have felt sad or miserable:

❏ Yes, most of the time
❏ Yes, quite often
❏ Not very often
❏ No, not at all

9 I have been so unhappy that I have been crying:

❏ Yes, most of the time
❏ Yes, quite often
❏ Only occasionally
❏ No, never

10 The thought of harming myself has occurred to me:

❏ Yes, quite often
❏ Sometimes
❏ Hardly ever
❏ Never

How the Scale Works

The Edinburgh Postnatal Depression Scale (EPDS) should be offered to all mums as a tool to asses where you are on the scale. It may be that you only score 0-7 points and this is fine, so unless things change this would be the end of EPDS for you. However, if you are feeling either a bit down or very low and depressed, the quiz will help to asses where you are on the scale, which is from 0-30 (with 30 being a very high score).

What your score means

0-7 means you are feeling fine, though understandably you can feel a little up and down with a new baby.

8-14 is borderline and your health visitor will come and see you again in less than six weeks to see how things are going.

15+ means you are showing some anxiety and depression. You can agree with the health visitor the action you'd like to take.

If you would like extra support to help you with anxiety or depression, some options might be:

- Agree when you'd like another visit from your health visitor in about a month's time.
- Have Listening Visits from your health visitor every few weeks to give you the opportunity to talk about things.
- Have a referral to community psychiatric nurse.
- Have a referral to your doctor for medication or a mental health service if that would help.

It is your choice what help and support you want – you can change your mind at any time or take the time to think it over and discuss it with your partner.

The Edinburgh Postnatal is just a tool to see where you are at on the anxiety and depression scale; it is NOT a test. This will not be seen in a negative way concerning the baby (I know it is a very common fear of new mums that someone will take their baby away; this would never happen as a result of doing this quiz). Do be honest; it is not a test of you as a mother, and no one will think you are a bad mum if you are feeling down. It is very common to be a bit down at some point following the birth of your baby. If you think about the overwhelming change and responsibilities you now have it is unsurprising that so many new mums have some feelings of depression or are just feeling a bit flat and out of sync. Your health visitor may suggest options for the help that is available for you. If you don't feel like you can talk to your health visitor then your doctor will also be able to offer help and support.

Some of the physical changes many new mums experience

It often seems that physical challenges resulting from having a baby seem to come when you feel least able to deal with them and have very little time for taking care of yourself. I've listed a few of the most common issues new mums face and some solutions to help get you feeling back on track. Be kind to yourself and don't expect too much of yourself on days when you feel tired or sore. Don't be embarrassed or worried about wasting people's time – your health matters and there are no silly questions when it comes to the well-being of you and your baby – for many women this is completely new territory and not what you expected from the early days of motherhood.

Bladder problems

It is quite common for mums to experience bladder problems (like a little bit of wee slipping out if you laugh or sneeze). The National Health Service offers a trained women's physiotherapist to help with this. Your health visitor or doctor can refer you and give you some pelvic floor exercises to do that will help tone things up a bit down there after giving birth. You usually get a leaflet on this in hospital or from your midwife or health visitor as well. If you are experiencing any problems, do tell someone; your six- to eight-week postnatal check-up with your doctor could also be a good opportunity to mention this or any other physical or emotional issues.

Stitches or tearing

Your body has done some very hard work in labour and delivery and you may have had stitches or a tear that needs time to heal. Your midwife in hospital and then at home will be the best person to discuss any concerns you have. If you are experiencing pain, discomfort or are concerned about the stitches, it is worth getting it properly checked by your midwife or doctor.

Many stitches are dissolvable but some stubbornly refuse to dissolve and cause discomfort, itching and soreness. Your midwife can check the healing for you and remove them if they have done their job and you've healed, even though the stitches may not have dissolved. Many women find that two to three drops of tea tree oil in a daily bath can help soothe things if you've had tearing and/or stitches. If you don't have a bath tub, applying very gentle pressure with warm (not hot) water from a hand-held shower can also be beneficial in soothing the perineal area, which you can dry with the warm setting on your hairdryer, as rubbing with a towel may only add to your discomfort. Wearing soft cotton knickers will not only be more comfortable but help keep the area as dry as possible.

Some women find they are still bleeding or have a dark red spotting of blood for several days before it darkens to brown and then to a straw-coloured discharge. This can be hard to deal with; finding the time to care for yourself when you have a new baby to take care of, combined with feeling fed up with the whole process, is a challenge for many mums after giving birth. Some women find it makes them feel unattractive or have some feelings of revulsion; this should not last for long, and if it persists for several weeks or months then do discuss these issues with your health visitor, doctor or the sexual health team at your local clinic.

Haemorrhoids and constipation

Constipation and haemorrhoids affect many mums and may have been a problem for you while you were pregnant. Haemorrhoids, often called piles, are swollen and enlarged veins in or around the anus. They can be very sore and itchy and very uncomfortable, and you may have a feeling of lumpiness or that your bowel still feels full even just after you've had a poo. You may pass a little blood when having a poo, especially if you are constipated, which often happens in the days after you've given birth. Tell your midwife or doctor if there is blood. You may need a laxative like Lactulose to soften your poo if you have constipation, and a health professional or pharmacist can advise on preparations to treat the haemorrhoids as well.

An ice pack may ease the pain and reduce swelling. You can fill an unused condom with cold water and freeze it to make a small ice pack that you can press against the sore area around the anus. A little more fibre in your diet and drinking water more frequently will help get things back to normal. You can take action to prevent constipation by having vegetable soup, fruit and vegetables as well as wholemeal bread in your diet as soon as you start eating again after delivery. Do ask for help as soon as you can, as both constipation and haemorrhoids are treatable and you needn't carry on in silence if problems persist. I know it can feel embarrassing but it's an everyday part of the job for health professionals and it is something a lot of new mothers experience.

Iron deficiency

Many women lose quite a substantial amount of blood during and following labour. Anaemia can be a problem for many mums especially in the months following the birth of your baby. You can check by looking at the lining of your eye: if it is very pale pink or grey pink you may well be anaemic and may need to take an iron supplement (red pink is the normal colour). Talk to your midwife or health visitor and have your haemoglobin checked with your doctor if needed and get advice on what would be the best iron supplement for you to take.

Sore breasts

In Chapter 1 (and in the A–Z section) you'll find more information on the problems women experience when breast-feeding and after birth, including treating sore and chapped nipples. If you are experiencing very sore or painful breasts, or blocked ducts or mastitis, it is important that you seek medical help from your midwife, health visitor or doctor as soon as you can.

Sex and your relationship with your partner

If you are in a relationship and are the main carer for your child, many women feel their partner doesn't understand how much their life has changed and how challenging it is to care for a baby all day and then all night. It can be good to share frustrations with other new mums, your own mum or sisters, but you don't want to be permanently resentful of your partner as it doesn't make for a happy baby or a happy family. Understanding the gap there seems to be in how men and women often perceive parenthood can be helpful in working out how to find solutions if you want more support from your partner.

Being responsible for your Little One 24 hours a day is a huge responsibility – give yourself credit for all you are doing and try not to be self-critical. Looking after your baby is wonderful in many ways, but it can create all sorts of anxieties – and everyone has anxieties no matter how calm they may appear on the outside. Sharing how you feel with your partner, parents or friends may help and reduce the burden. In meeting your baby's physical and emotional needs you are doing the most important thing in any society: raising a happy and well-adjusted child who can reach their potential. It's not easy – it may well be the hardest thing you ever do – but the rewards are immense and there is so much joy in seeing your baby grow and develop into a special person that you both created. It can be a time that really helps you grow together as a couple, but it takes teamwork.

He doesn't know what to do

If you feel your concerns are being dismissed as trivial by your partner it can often be because your partner is at a loss to know what to do themselves. Many men will say they 'want you back the way you used to be', which can feel like a real slap in the face. If your partner wants to see you like your old self, you're more likely to be happy if they acknowledge your feelings and concerns. Some men don't realise that a few understanding words or a hug

can make all the difference – it is often the little daily signs of consideration and affection we need to raise self-esteem. It is knowing that both of you are in this together and that having a baby is a life-changing achievement which is bound to feel overwhelming at times for both of you. A little kindness goes a long way.

I have spoken to many women who feel they are run off their feet and doing all the work caring for the new baby, whilst at the same time their partner has his own unexpressed feelings of rejection. New dads often talk about thinking they are a bit useless and no longer needed now their partner has *her baby*. It usually takes longer for men to find their role, and the more involved dads become, the more opportunity they have for finding what their strengths are in parenting and homemaking.

Life can start to feel more demanding around the 6–12 months stage; all the help and support mums often get with a new baby has usually by now evaporated. Often you'll have big decisions to make about childcare, work and finance. Many women feel

like they're expected to work, take care of the house and a now very mobile baby who requires feeds, meals, playtime, nap times, nappy changes, washing and creates endless mess. If you do start to feel like you are trapped or that all the work falls to you and you want more support, then talk about your feelings. This can be tricky with a partner, and the temptation is to do a big list of all you are doing, which often results in an argument as partners feel they are being blamed. It may help if you describe the situation and how it makes you feel, then ask your partner how they feel and how they might be able to support you and the relationship.

Having sex again after having a baby

After you have a baby so many things change: your relationship and how you feel about being a mum, how you feel about your body and how you feel about your partner. Mums and dads can still be great lovers, though (it's just finding the time and energy to do it!). You may be really looking forward to getting the all-clear to resume sexual activity again after the birth of your baby, or it may be the last thing on your mind for quite some time. There is no right or wrong way to feel, and you have to be true to yourself. One thing I've noticed is that women are more likely to want to be intimate with a man who is sharing the trials and joys of parenthood with her than a man conspicuous by his absence when it comes to caring for the baby.

Having sex again for the first time can be a bit daunting. For some women it's reminiscent of losing their virginity all over again, and as we know that can be a good or a bad experience. Some couples are hesitant about resuming a full sex life due to fear of another pregnancy. It might be you have less libido, and understandably women who have had a traumatic delivery often have a great reluctance to have sex again. I'd suggest taking things gently and slowly to start with, so that you're not putting too much pressure on each other. Some women are physically and emotionally ready to resume sex again after six weeks, but every woman is different and in my experience many women aren't ready to have sex again for several more weeks or even several months following the birth.

During sex if anything is painful, stop right away and give

it several days to a week before you try again. If the pain doesn't go away, talk to your health visitor or doctor. Some women not only take longer to heal but are not emotionally ready to have sex again for some time after giving birth, and a partner needs to respect that. If you want to, there are other things you can both enjoy if penetrative sex is off the agenda for a while. Just do what you want to do, and what feels right for both of you. If you and your partner communicate, and find the space and time that works for you both, it can be a really special time to rediscover each other during those weekend afternoons when your baby is having a nap – skip the supermarket (get the groceries delivered instead) and have some 'us' time.

If you feel that you don't want to have sex with your partner, it is worth taking the time to consider the effect this will have on him. It is very likely that frequent rebuffs to his sexual advances will leave him feeling rejected, and that you no longer want him now you have your baby (and worth considering for yourself if this is true?). You are both entitled to your thoughts and feeling and it is good to try and see the situation from the other person's point of view.

You have the right not to have sex, but your partner has the right to his feelings, too. I've spoken to mothers who have told me they are just too exhausted to even think of sex after having a baby; all they want is some sleep and a hot meal. Some new mothers have told me of their fear of having sex again. It is very common for women (and men!) to be worried about sex being painful or that it will result in pregnancy.

It may be that you don't know yourself why you don't want to have sex, and feel embarrassed or uncertain about discussing these complex emotions with your partner in case it all comes out wrong and results in an argument. I've found that choosing the right time to have these conversations makes a big difference to the outcome. If a woman is faced with an unwanted sexual advance from her partner and chooses this moment to list the reasons she doesn't want to have sex with him, neither of them is going to get very far. If you've just turned your partner down, reassure him that you really love him but aren't ready for sex at the moment. Many women need to talk about having sex again before they do it. It might be a non-emotionally charged chat over coffee or on a walk will turn out a bit better than at midnight. It is not an easy situation, and rarely resolved immediately, but keep talking and listening to each other if you can, as open lines of communication will help your understanding of each other and build trust.

Sometimes it's useful to have a chance to discuss your feelings with a health professional who has to keep the conversation private and confidential. This could be your health visitor or doctor. If you feel the situation is getting serious and you need specialist help, a relationship/sex therapist may be worth asking about. The health visitor or sexual health clinic could do this referral for both of you, or just for you if your partner doesn't want to go. Another option is to contact Relate, the UK charity that offers relationship counselling. For many couples any problems they experience after the birth of their baby will be of short duration and they do not need any help from external source, though it is there if you want it.

I remember when ... I bumped into a mum whom I'd visited from the time when her first baby was ten days old till her third baby went to primary school. She told me that the first time I ever visited her and her husband with their new baby, her husband was standing behind my chair mouthing at her, 'Ask her when we can have sex?' I wasn't aware of this at the time, and when I thought back on it I did wonder why she sighed such a huge sigh of relief when I asked if they had any questions about sex. It reminded me how important it is to give parents an opportunity not only to discuss contraceptive choices but to give them the time to talk about their relationship and sex if it's something they want to do. The more I've had these conversations over the years, the more I've realised just saying it's usually OK after six to eight weeks really isn't giving couples the information they need and is just a very rough guideline, not a target.

You're a Normal New Mum if You...

1. Feel up one minute and down the next. (If the downs get too frequent or extreme, do get some help.)

2. Take a bit of time to adjust to life as a mum. Be kind to yourself and give yourself credit for the good things I know you are already doing.

3. Don't want to go to every group and activity you're told about. Only do the things you want to do – this is your time with your new baby; spend it how you like.

4. Want a little bit of time for yourself and with your partner. If the opportunity arises for a few hours' break to get a meal or go for a walk and recharge your batteries, take it.

5. Still crave those intimate moments with your partner. Opportunities for romance can be few and far between with a new baby, but being kind to each other and affectionate is definitely do-able and beneficial to your whole family.

6. Still have your own emotional and physical needs. Being clear about the support you need to ensure you get to eat, wash and sleep as well will help you better meet the needs of your baby.

7. Take up offers of help (they soon dry up!). If meals, cleaning services or offers to nip to the shops are made, take them – you've got enough to do.

8. Aren't a perfect mother ... because there is no such person! If you are a bit of a perfectionist by nature, just prioritise the essentials (dust will always be there, your new baby is growing fast – enjoy them).

5

Finding Your Role as a New Dad and Supporting Your Partner

Your life has changed forever literally overnight. You might wonder how caring for one tiny person seems to take all day and all night. You may feel you've completely taken to parenthood and aren't anxious about what to do and not to do, but many of us learn on the job and sometimes you don't want an audience because it can feel like everyone is judging your ability to be a good parent. Have you ever noticed when it comes to babies, practically everyone has an opinion, whether you want to hear it or not?

Dads come to parenthood without the benefits of changes to their body that women experience and with no outer sign that they are going to become a parent. The emphasis, quite naturally, is on the health and well-being of mother and baby. As the father, you are the person who probably most desires a safe pregnancy and delivery of a healthy baby and the well-being of your partner. Pregnancy is an anxious time for you both, and most dads are secondary to the process of antenatal appointments and classes. Keep in mind that your partner really needs your support and strength, not just in pregnancy and labour, but even more so in the first few months after your baby is born.

You may have seen the birth of your baby and found it a moving and wonderful experience. Many men feel very fearful for their partner and baby during the process of labour, and it is a moment of huge relief and pride when your child is safely delivered. Mums often say that although labour is very painful and traumatic in many ways, they eventually forget some of the process, while you may feel you remember it all and feel a little traumatised yourself, but as it was your partner's pain and experience it is understandable that your experience does come second. Nevertheless, you may have found labour was dramatic and feel quite stirred up by it, and mostly no one acknowledges this so there can be feelings that are very mixed up for you as well in the first days and weeks after the birth.

Involved, committed and caring fathers make a huge difference to the health and well-being of both mothers and babies; couples working together as a team is one of the reasons that this is the best generation of parents there has ever been.

Trust Yourself

Tell Your Partner How You Feel about Her

Many men have even greater love and admiration for their partner once she becomes a mother, and it is really important you tell her that, not once or twice but often. A few kind words, a hug and a no-strings-attached kiss can really help your partner to feel appreciated.

For your baby and your family to be happy it is vital that you play a full part in the care and upbringing of your child, but sometimes it can be bewildering to know what to do for the best. The responsibilities can seem overwhelming and it is not always easy to see how you can help, even when you want to so much, and be the best dad you can be.

Trust Yourself

Set Some Boundaries
Be specific about when it'll be OK for people to visit: say something like, 'You're very welcome. If you'd like to pop in for a coffee and to say hello between 3-4 pm on Thursday, that would be great.' Really good guests will bring cake with them.

Protect your partner by managing visitors

As soon as your baby is born one of the ways you can help your family is by managing the amount of family, friends and neighbours who want to see your Little One. It is to be expected that there may be days when having visitors is too much for you and your partner, even if you have a fantastic support network of family and friends and feel comfortable about having guests. Whatever your partner wants on the day is usually the best thing to do, even if you feel you'll be disappointing people. In the early days, don't be worried about asking for some privacy and calm in your home as you adjust to family life – good friends and relations will always understand. Wanting a little time alone to adapt to parenthood and enjoy this precious time isn't selfish, it makes complete sense.

Your role in the first weeks is to be the gatekeeper. Neither of you wants people to be knocking on your door when you've just got the baby to sleep and are ready for some much-needed shut-eye yourself. As the gate-keeper you can answer the calls, emails and texts on behalf of your partner and arrange times for people to visit. It may be easier for you rather than your partner to say, 'No, we

aren't ready for visitors just yet.' Or, if you do want people to stop by, make it clear when and for how long they can stay and give them some friendly hints when it's time to go.

Don't be afraid to cancel. If you're having a difficult day and your partner says she really can't face visitors, then just tell people it's not a good time. Keep tabs on how she's feeling: life with a new baby can leave you being on top of the world one minute and in tears the next. So, whether you decide people can stop by every other day, three times a week, or once a week – suit yourselves.

Entertaining people takes a lot of preparation. Your partner will need to be well nourished because you'll have noticed the day mainly consists of feeding, feeding, feeding. If funds allow, get your shopping delivered so that's one thing less to do. Food that's easy to warm up is a blessing, and you're going to need that energy-giving, nourishing food now more than ever.

Visitor Checklist

If friends and family want to help out, let them know that a homemade stew, lasagne or a cake would be very welcome. It'll give you the time you need to focus on taking care of your baby and yourself if you're not having to worry about food.

❑ Be specific about when and for how long you want visitors.

❑ Put yourselves first. Whatever you want to do is the right thing to do.

❑ Accept offers of home-cooked meals, or do an online shop.

Dads sometimes feel a bit pushed out

Having a baby does change everything, and some dads feel a bit pushed out or redundant. You may think that you are not as good at caring for the baby or knowing what to do next. Don't worry about it if the baby's nappy is a bit wonky or you feel nervous about bathing your precious new Little One; just have a go and be involved from the off.

If you try to do your bit without asking what to do all the time and show you are more than capable of adapting to your new situation as things come up, it will boost your and your partner's confidence in working together as a team. Being responsive, caring and willing to do your bit means you are halfway there; the rest is just practice, and you'll learn something new every day. Your partner and baby will benefit hugely the more you are involved; dads can bring such fun, laughter and strength by sharing the responsibility of caring for their Little One.

It can seem like new mums are on top of the world with joy one minute and feeling quite low and lost the next. Reassure her that you're there for her, and that you think she's doing a really amazing job. I know sometimes it feels like you take all the flack and nothing you do is right, but this phase of adjusting to life with a new baby is soon over, though I know it doesn't feel like that at the time. Most new mums' lives are totally consumed by feeding, feeding, feeding. It completely dominates her life in the first few months, and there is no break from it. It will be some time before she has any baby-free time at all, and you may get to go to work and leave the responsibilities of parenthood be-

> ## Trust Yourself
>
> ### Be a Super Daddy
> Doing the housework, washing, shopping and meals (or roping in grandparents and friends to lend a hand as well) will give your partner the chance to get some rest when she isn't looking after the baby.

hind you for a few hours even though you might not have the most stress-free job in the world yourself and miss your baby and partner, and would much rather be at home with them.

Are you a hunter-gatherer dad?

Men's and women's priorities after having a baby are often slightly out of sync, too. Many new fathers feel an overwhelming need to work their socks off to support their new family, and seem to be working harder than ever to provide – it's a hunter-gatherer thing, maybe! But many women would much rather have their partner at home to help. To ensure you are both on the same page and appreciate the effort you are both making to provide a loving, secure and happy home for your baby, it is important to have a calm, non-accusatory discussion about where your priorities are and recognise the contribution each of you makes.

When you get home from work you may find your partner is desperate for you to take the baby off her hands just so she can be physically free and get a shower, some food or some sleep. Even if you've had a hard day and are tired and want a bit of time for relaxation, do not say this, as it is unlikely to go down well with your partner! Also stay well clear of remarks like, 'What have you been doing all day?' if you want to avoid a row. For your

partner, saying things like this implies it is easy being at home with the baby – when taking care of a baby is probably the most physically and emotionally demanding thing she will ever do. Resentment can easily build that you don't understand how hard things are for her, and that your contribution is never as great as hers.

If you are in any doubt about this, or would like to gain a greater insight into what your partner is experiencing, then offer to look after the baby all on your own when your baby is ready for a bit of separation from mum. Ask your partner to give you some expressed breast milk or make up the formula yourself if you are bottle feeding, and take care of the baby for a day or even half a day without any help from anyone. It'll give you a better insight into her world and a chance to see if you can also do all the daily tasks she does as well (like cleaning and shopping or making a phone call, even). Staying at home is not the easy option if you are properly meeting all your baby's physical and emotional needs, and it's important for your partner that you show you recognise this.

Let's talk about sex!

Since your baby arrived have you noticed a change in your relationship with your partner? Whether you expected things to be different or not, it is understandable that the arrival of an extra person in your household will inevitably change the dynamics of your relationship. Just think if you had a relative, friend or lodger move in with you, things would be different – so your new baby, although very welcome, will change some things about you both. The bottom line is your world and the way you perceive it alter when you have a baby. It is really worth giving some thought to how things have changed and how you and your partner will adapt and enjoy life with each other and the new baby.

Just because you are parents, it doesn't mean that being a couple and enjoying a sex life together is a thing of the past; it's just that after having a baby, romance isn't always uppermost in people's minds. For many couples the arrival of your baby can mean there is very little time, if any, for sex, and some men do feel a bit redundant once their partner has *her baby*.

On a purely biological note, a woman is programmed by nature to reproduce, and once she has the baby she craves and has longed for, nature no longer needs the man, for a while. That does not mean your partner doesn't need or want you, but she may have these unconscious instincts for a short time after having a baby. I think our early forebears were so intent on the survival of the infant that all the attention and protection

Five Ways to Be a Positive Partner

1 Help with the baby and enjoy being a dad.

2 Ask about her feelings and be honest about yours.

3 Build up to sex slowly; don't just be affectionate with hugs and kisses when you want to have sex.

4 Give your partner some time on her own while you look after the baby.

5 Make sure she knows how much you love her and that you still find her attractive.

went towards the baby; dinner and a movie followed by coffee and dessert weren't on the menu. This is just an explanation of what may be behind the lack of libido for women following childbirth, but if you both want to you can get your sex life back on track.

When two people put the needs of their baby first it really does make for happy babies. That does not mean men and women have equal lives, though. A woman's world changes completely when she has a baby, she has very little option on this, but most men do; though I'm happy to say more and more dads are working as a team with their partner. The more positive involvement dads have, the happier families are. Being involved in your baby's life right from the start is like nothing else you will ever experience, and it can take your relationship with your partner to new levels of love and intimacy if you do it together.

It is normal to want to have sex with your partner

There is nothing wrong or unfair about wanting a sex life, and some women are physically and emotionally ready to start exploring their sexual side six weeks or thereabouts after birth. But your partner may not be physically and emotionally ready so soon after giving birth. Showing frustration or anger about lack of sex will not help her come round any faster, and could put her off sex completely. Your partner may not want to have sex, but it won't be because she doesn't love you any more, though it may feel you are rather low on the agenda at the moment.

It is perfectly normal to want to resume your sex life as an important part of your relationship. Just don't expect too much too soon. Listen to your partner and act on what she tells you. Whilst intercourse may be off the menu for a while, your wife may be open to other ways of meeting both your sexual needs. You as a couple need to have a frank and open talk, again without being reproachful or getting annoyed or angry about your sexual needs and hers (or possibly lack of need) to see how both of you can resolve this.

If your partner is breastfeeding her breasts may be temporarily off-limits and you'll need to respect that. Again, this will not be forever, but it can seem as if it is a rejection of you and your needs, and even when one knows this is not true from an intellectual perspective it can hurt and frustrate you, and it would be strange if you didn't have some feelings of rejection. If your partner is dreading a sexual advance she may repel any physical affection from you if she sees it as a signal of your desire for sex; this can be on an unconscious level for both of you and lead to feelings of rejection and frustration on both sides.

It is worth remembering that in giving birth a woman's body can be physically traumatised. The fear of sex being painful or the fear of getting pregnant again can result in a lack of libido and she may be unwilling to get back to your previous sex life. Nature does play a part in this, and some women say that although their affection and love for their husband is as strong, if not stronger, than before they became parents, they are too exhausted to even think about sex. This is usually only during the first few weeks or months, and usually a woman's desire to have sex will return at some stage. It is worth trying to discuss this, but as we've said choose your moment and try not to make it an accusation. It may help to start with affection, just a hug or a kiss on her brow or head to show your love for her without the expectation that this will lead to sex.

Trust Yourself

1st and 2nd Base

You don't have to go all the way! For many women it is getting a hug, a kiss, a soft touch or a smile that makes them feel loved. Small signs of affection can really boost energy levels and help you both to feel reconnected and secure.

Before you begin a conversation about your relationship and having sex it would help to have an idea of what to say. Start with the positive: tell her how happy you are to be a dad and that you are proud of her and your baby. Maybe just say you understand that your sex life needs to be secondary to the baby's needs right now but that your love and desire for her are still the same and that you know that your love will be strengthened by your joint love for your baby.

What to Do (and Not to Do) if You Want to Have Sex Again

1. **Pick the right time and place** to talk about how she feels about having sex. (For example, not when she's tired or upset or in the middle of something, and definitely not when you are hoping to have sex!)

2. **Avoid clumsy attempts to initiate sex** without any lead-in or discussion. Make sure you have an insight into how she feels by listening to her and taking on board her fears, concerns ... or even desires!

3. **When you give her a cuddle or a kiss, do not expect it to lead to sex.** Be affectionate because you love her, not because you are hoping it will lead to sex, or you may find your partner doesn't want any physical contact at all.

4. **Be honest about your own feelings.** If you are feeling pushed out or rejected, talk about why you feel this way calmly. Talking about feelings without being accusatory, angry, reproachful or censorious takes practice ... it is very hard to be fair, especially when we are feeling rejected.

5. **Make sure you partner knows you still love her and find her attractive.** Some women's physical and sexual confidence can take a bit of a dip after pregnancy and birth.

Many women respond more to words and caring than sexual advances, and in showing your strength of love and willingness to wait it may help to rekindle feelings of love and desire in her for you.

Asking her about how she feels about having sex again is a way for you to understand what is holding her back. You need to be ready to listen to her, to be open about your own feelings and be prepared that you might not get the response you were hoping for. I've listed a few suggestions on how to get the conversation started.

Having a new baby can be tough for you as well as for your partner, and physical exhaustion takes its toll on both of you. Babies need their dads as well as their mums, and you will find reserves of strength and maturity that you didn't know you had. You may find a confidential chat with a friend, your dad or uncle will help, and show that it is normal for things to be a bit turbulent after having a baby. Enjoy your baby and your relationship and feel justifiable pride in all your achievements in parenting and being a brilliant dad. This is your opportunity to build a closer relationship with your partner as well as with your baby.

Trust Yourself Checklist

Here are a few positive acknowledgements so you can trust that you are doing everything you can to look after yourself, your baby and your partner.

❑ After having a baby emotions run high. This is normal and natural, but if things start to feel unbearable, seek help.

❑ It's really important for new mums to look after themselves. Physical and emotional changes are to be expected, and there is help should you need it.

❑ Raising a happy, well-adjusted baby isn't easy, but it is the most important thing we can do in any society.

❑ Mums and dads will have a happier time if they work together as a team and support each other.

❑ Listen to your partner. It is the listening, not the talking, that is often the most challenging part of good communication (if you are thinking about what you are going to say next, you aren't really listening!).

6

Five Things You Can Do to Have a Happy Baby – and Understanding Their Development

Meeting your baby's emotional needs is a crucial component to happiness, yet is often overlooked as people tend to talk more about milestones. Watching your baby grow and develop is such a joy, and it is so much more than walking and talking. The unique relationship you develop with your child will be founded in your first year with your Little One and is full of opportunities for fun and laughter. The pressure some parents feel that their baby should be rolling over at a certain stage or feeding themselves can come from the expectations other people often have; that a child should crawl at a particular month or start to babble by a set age. Without realising it comparisons are made, and this can create unnecessary anxiety; most children develop at their own pace and your child has their own path to follow. More often than not parents are meeting many of their baby's needs unconsciously and instinctively, but it can be helpful to recognise the broad areas of need that will make your baby feel loved. Nearly all parents know a baby needs to be loved, but as well as this it is vital your child also feels secure.

My approach for creating emotional security is based largely on the work of Dr Mia Kellmer Pringle who founded the National Children's Bureau. My philosophy is that when you meet your child's emotional needs as well as their physical needs, all your hard work will be rewarded with a happy and well-attached baby. Our understanding of growth and development is drawn from the pioneering work of Dr Mary Sheridan. She was a paediatrician who identified the areas of a baby's development and how to observe and record these milestones. She also developed what to do in the case of any area of problem or delay in development, and it is worth remembering that she said that doctors should, 'Listen to mother's suspicions about any concern about her baby because she is usually right.' Wise words indeed! The age ranges are just for broad reference and are not targets. It is nice to know your baby has reached another stage of their development, but if you have any concerns always talk to your health visitor or doctor, either at your baby's health checks or by making an appointment.

Growth relates to the increasing size of your baby, usually by measuring your Little One's weight, height and head circumference and plotting these on a graph called a percentile chart which is usually recorded by a health visitor. Development milestones note the way your baby's senses, movement, speech and language and cognitive skills are developing.

The Five Emotional Needs of Children

The building blocks for positive parenting that create a happy child in their first year are:

1. Love;
2. Security;
3. Praise and recognition;
4. New experiences; and
5. Responsibility and discipline

I remember when ... I was a newly qualified health visitor in the mid-1970s in rural Kent. Dr Mia Kellmer Pringle came to speak to our health professionals' quarterly meeting about her work and her book *The Emotional Needs of Children*. On a cold winter's evening in the village hall I listened, enraptured, as she told us about how, though most parents met children's practical needs and did love their children, they didn't show it or put a high value on their child's emotional well-being. She told us that the need for love and security was as important to the psyche as food and drink is to the body. She made a lasting, deep impression on me but I was unaware of how important her ideas were at the time and how much they would influence the rest of my career. At my earliest opportunity I read her book and realised that feeling loved, secure, receiving praise and recognition and having responsibility were crucial to all human beings' happiness. As the years went on saw first hand that new experiences were also an important factor in how parents nurture their Little Ones.

1. Love

Today's parents are, more often than not, a long way away from past generations of parents who mostly loved their children but didn't always show it. Many parents and grandparents in the last century didn't express their love for their children, and it wasn't the norm to show your baby how much you loved them on a daily basis with words of love and encouragement, cuddles and kisses. If your parents *were* affectionate, positive people and you felt very much at the centre of their lives, then you'll know what an amazing, special and powerful feeling this is.

In the past parents often didn't show love and sympathy in the same way because they believed that quickly attending to a crying or distressed baby would 'spoil' the child. Happily, we now know that the reverse of this is true, and ensuring your baby feels loved is the most important thing any parent can do. It is balancing your baby's needs with your own and the rest of your family that is tricky. Mums do have their own needs as well, and you can't have a happy baby without a happy mummy.

Mums and dads often show their love in different ways

Dads play a crucial part in loving the baby, too, though how they show that love can be different. Dads often express their love by playing with or entertaining the baby. They need to have space and time to find their own path and be able to express their own feelings of love, which develop over time. Dads have not had the advantage of a baby developing over nine months inside them and the physical process of giving birth that a mother experiences, but recognising the love you each give your child is a very positive thing to do.

Kisses, cuddles, play and loving touches often come naturally to a lot of parents, but if that wasn't how you were raised sometimes it does take a bit of conscious effort to do things differently and show how much you love your baby every day. Often parents experience some of their happiest moments together during playtime. Smiling and laughing are just lovely; they set up two-way communication with your Little One. Listening to your baby and leaving a gap for a response is a worthwhile habit to get into, as before you know it your baby will soon make little noises when you are talking to them and it is amazing to see your baby start to interact with you. From their earliest days your baby can benefit by listening to you read to them and looking at the pictures in books. It becomes a cornerstone in their childhood days that helps them to feel loved and secure as well as helping to develop their speech and language skills. It gives them the opportunity and confidence to get involved and be a member of your family.

As long as a baby has one parent or caregiver to whom that baby's care, happiness and development is paramount, it is my belief that the baby will grow up to be a happy, well-contented individual. Not every baby will have two parents or be raised by their biological parents, but they can grow to be just as happy and well-balanced as any other child. One loving person can provide all a baby needs, but it is a very big challenge to that one parent, and they will need support from other sources.

If you've adopted a baby, all the preparation and waiting that you have done before your Little One came into your lives is good preparation and demonstrates your unconditional and overwhelming love for your new baby. The sooner a baby is with their adoptive parents, the better opportunity they have to make their Little One feel loved every day and to develop attachment.

It's important for all babies to have the opportunity to get to know their carer's face and become familiar with their surroundings from their earliest days. You may have noticed babies are fascinated by faces. Very soon they start to look about them and be really interested in their home and familiar places. They'll soon start to follow a conversation and recognise when something is going to happen, like a feed, and make pleased gurgling noises. From the start you can make your baby part of the conversation by narrating what's happening, talking to them and leaving that gap for their response.

As they grow, give them the opportunity to make choices and treat them with respect and equality.

Knowing you are loved changes everything

Love is the foundation building block on which everything else is dependent. For a child to realise and actualise their potential in life and to become a well-balanced, happy and considerate person, they need to know they are loved every single day. There is no true attachment without an all-encompassing love for your baby – you couldn't give yourself so willingly to your child without it. Once your baby is born, a parent feels like the love they have for their baby is like no other love; it is unconditional and it is very one-sided – because the baby has no way of being reciprocal. As your Little One grows they will learn from you how to be a considerate, loving person, who can balance their needs with the needs of others.

2. Security

A lot of baby care focuses on the practical needs of your baby, but meeting your child's emotional needs is just as important because whether or not a child has a strong attachment to their parent or carer is life-altering; it is what makes you feel secure in yourself and those around you. The changes you made in your life while you were waiting for your baby are all part of the preparation for parenthood; so, rest assured the connection you have with your child started before they were even born – I'm sure you are already well on the way to having a secure, well-attached and loving relationship with your baby.

That sounds a bit scary, as if you have to be the perfect parent, but you will be doing so much to achieve attachment every single day you won't even realise you are already doing it. When your newborn baby gazes at you intensely and listens to your voice (which they often recognise immediately from birth, having heard it when in the womb), you are building a stronger attachment by making them the centre of your life and creating a home that is both loving and secure.

Even when they are tiny your baby may have a favourite tune. If you sang to them or played certain

music during pregnancy, it often has a calming effect on a baby because it is familiar and associated with being safe and warm and snug. Even your animated body language and hand movements during a simple song like 'Incy Wincey Spider' or 'Twinkle, Twinkle Little Star' soon becomes filled with familiar movements and sounds that reassure, comfort, distract and amuse your Little One. Babies soon learn to make squealing noises of delight when they see you, and you may notice your Little One sometimes goes quiet at the sound of your and your partner's voices. Familiar sounds regularly heard as part of the fabric of their day all help to make your baby feel secure. By around nine months this ability to recognise and respond will develop into speech, showing their understanding, delight or annoyance verbally without only having the option of crying.

Those familiar games and songs will become more interactive and they'll start to join in and then to initiate actions like waving bye-bye or playing 'Peepo'. This is the interweaving of the full spectrum of their emotional, physical and intellectual development that helps them to interpret themselves and the world and people around them.

Meeting your baby's emotional needs swiftly is not spoiling them

Every day you will be working to meet your baby's physical and emotional needs. One of the ways you show your love for your baby is by making them feel secure and being consistent in the way you behave with your Little One. A swift response to your baby will not spoil them but help them develop a feeling of security as they realise someone is on hand to meet their needs and provide comfort, love and reassurance when they are distressed.

You will not be spoiling your baby by meeting their emotional needs; in fact, I think it is impossible to spoil a baby by loving them and putting them first – it is exactly what they need, and if this is what you try and practise each day, then you are a fabulous parent.

Putting them first isn't about letting your growing baby have all their own way all the time, but it is about being there for them when they need you, whether that's for a cuddle, to make them laugh, to tell them how wonderful they are, feeding them, changing a nappy or to taking them out of harm's way when they are crawling towards the plug socket – you are setting both physical and emotional boundaries to keep them safe and sound and happy.

Attachment isn't always easy

When your baby is born it's all about feeding, feeding, feeding; then as they grow it's all weaning, weaning, weaning. You'll notice as your Little One grows life is all about attachment, attachment, attachment! Though it is wonderful to make your baby feel secure, it is more demanding on you because an attached baby demands more from their parents. There are just a few babies who have an almost permanent happy disposition and rarely show any distress, so if this is your Little One's temperament, just be happy, it doesn't mean they are not attached to you; they just have a jolly, robust outlook.

You'll notice the signs your baby is developing attachment when they get upset if you are out of sight even for just a few minutes. Your Little One wants to be near you because it makes them feel secure, especially if they are hungry, tired or having teething pain – they just need that extra bit of reassurance. Distracting them with a game, a little TV or some forgotten toys will give you the opportunity to get their lunch ready, make a phone call or go to the loo without having to hear crying while you do it.

This constant need for you is all part of their growing sense of attachment, and they will soon be comforted by another caregiver or you when you get back (rest assured that a few minutes' separation won't do them any harm – you can't be

Babies Can't Wait

It is more likely that a swift response to your Little One will teach and show them that they are loved and wanted, and lead to a loved, secure and HAPPY BABY.

in their eye-line all the time!). Your baby has to realise for themselves that Mummy will come back when you leave the room or go away – this, too, draws on your reserves of patience and perseverance. It may not feel like it, but it's actually a really good sign, as it shows your baby is well attached to you. See it as a compliment to your parenting.

When only Mummy will do

You'll find it is often only you who can bring your baby comfort by being close to them, with your smell, your voice, the rise and fall of your breathing and your heartbeat. All these things help your baby to feel secure because they know you are near. Even during the everyday tasks like washing or applying cream to their skin, it is this attention and the sensation of touch that contribute to the closeness your baby feels for you (another good reason for Dad to get in on the act with bathing and nappy-changing early on!). We can see, then, that attachment is all part of the things you do for your baby and how you show your care and love for them – it's the way that you do it that makes the difference. Building a secure and rewarding relationship and having a happy baby, mum and dad is so important, not just for the early days but for life-long happy relationships. There are always challenges and setbacks when raising children, but the firm foundations you lay in these early years will most certainly lead to a wonderful closeness that will endure all your life.

For many mums or the person who is the main carer, babies will go through a period where they will cling to you and be reluctant to go to anyone else. They become uncertain about new or even familiar people. It may take 10 or 15 minutes until they are happy to interact with other people; just follow your baby's lead.

Trust Yourself

A Little Relaxation Goes a Long Way

If you need to leave your LO and you think they are going to start crying, take a few minutes to prepare yourself. Drop your shoulders, close your eyes and take ten slow, deep breaths in and out. The less anxious you are, the better you'll both do.

Getting everyone involved in a game is a good way to make them at ease with others so you can take a step back. It's understandable that your baby may want you all the time, but often they can't have this for practical reasons *and* you need a break too.

Does every day need to be the same?

Babies do like the familiar, but this does not mean you should follow a strict regime to make every day the same. It is your consistency in behaviour and understanding that help your Little One feel secure, not doing exactly the same things in the same way every day – in fact babies love new experiences and a little bit of variety.

Having a mini-routine or general plan for your day can help you ensure you know what is needed to meet your baby's needs. Things adjust and change all the time with a baby, so creating your own flexible schedule for the day rather than trying to fit in with someone else's often means there will be no tears before bedtime for you both. Try not to expect too much from yourselves; some days you'll be up for things and others you won't, and there's nothing wrong with that.

Routines are very changeable as you continually adapt your day to meet your baby's needs as they grow and develop, and it is this that helps your baby to feel secure. It is getting what they want when they need it: whether they feed at 11 am or 12 pm makes no difference to them; they don't know what time it is. Just do what feels right for you and your baby.

It is your calm, loving and consistent approach that will give your Little One the sense of security they need. It's not that you'll know automatically what to do in every situation (and you can't plan for everything), but following your gut feeling will almost certainly be best for both of you.

Should I leave my baby to cry?

It is important to recognise that all babies cry and sometimes from four to six months, or even earlier, babies start to test their boundaries as their attachment to their mother is growing and developing. Your Little One will begin to realise when you have left the room and sometimes they'll continue playing and other times they'll start to wail before you even take a couple of steps.

It is a sign your Little One is getting very attached to you if some days they are reluctant to let go of you at nap time or bedtime as they don't want to be separated, or they start having to have you within touching distance and want a fistful of your clothing or hair to hold on to. This can start very early and it is common from six to seven months onwards and lasts throughout the early years. It can be intense, very trying and a source of anxiety for many parents.

If they are crying at nap time, trust yourself on whether it feels like a grump or whether they are in distress and need comforting. It'll take about five minutes or so for your baby to grump themselves off to sleep, and whether you stay in the room or leave the room is up to you. Dim the lights, make them warm and secure and be near them as they take a few moments to grump and settle. If they aren't asleep after five to ten minutes but seem content and settled you can leave it a little longer if you want to. If you feel they are still hungry or just want a bit of extra comfort, do what feels right for you. If your baby is starting to get very fractious, soothe them and, when they are calm, try and settle them again. Be aware that most babies won't take to this the first time; it takes practice for both of you.

If your baby is really wailing, leaving them to cry it out will not achieve anything much for either of you. Some babies will eventually fall asleep through sheer exhaustion, but the consequence is the effect on the love and security they feel. So if you want to pick your baby up and comfort them, do just that. You know your child best. They aren't going to follow a rulebook; they are a person with the same feelings as you and me.

It might be a little bit of trial and error to find the techniques and coping strategies that feel right for you. Don't be too hard on yourself; some days you'll be calmer than others, depending on how much sleep you've had and whether you've had enough food and drink. Take each day as it comes; if your baby in very fractious, teething and feeling generally grumpy, often closeness is all they want, and if you are able to be there for them that's great, but some days you won't and someone else will need to care for them. As long as that person is caring, comforting and meets your baby's needs, it will not do your baby any harm at all. We all have to find ways of caring for our children in a way that feels right for us and is realistic to our personal circumstances. It is, though, a really good thing that your baby is well attached to you (even though it can sometimes feel like a burden), and another time when practising patience and perseverance is going to be what gets you through.

Is my older baby just attention-seeking?

Newborn babies always need a swift response, but older babies do cry and get worked up when they are looking for sympathy, not just when they are hungry, tired, feeling unwell or need their nappy changed. It is understandable they frequently want a bit of sympathy – attachment is often developing at a time when babies start to get really distressed with teething pain, are getting rather mobile and keep toppling over, and learning to hand-feed. That's a lot of stuff going on.

The good news is as they get older they'll have more ways to communicate their feelings and needs besides crying. You'll soon be talking their language, whether that's pointing, babbling or pulling themselves up to get something for themselves. Most of the time you'll be able to read whether their protesting is all a storm in a teacup or whether they are in need of some one-on-one time and lots of TLC – especially if their sudden bad-temperedness is out of character and you haven't been able to put them down all day.

All babies will cry no matter how dedicated a parent they have, and it is normal for their bottom lip to quiver and for them to do little protest cries when they get older. Just meet it with the level of sympathy and consideration you think it needs. There will be times when your baby is just attention-seeking. It is normal and natural and important for their development and their survival that your child has your attention.

Should my baby sleep in my bedroom?

Night-time is often when babies need extra attention to help them feel secure. When they are first born it is a good idea to have your baby near you. If space allows, having your baby in their crib in your room is good for both of you. (Check out

Chapter 3 for more infor- mation.) From six months a lot of mums move babies into a room of their own, to give both mother and baby a better night's sleep, but you may feel that you would prefer to keep your baby in the same room up until their first or second birthday, and that is absolutely fine too. It is a personal decision; no one should tell you when or when not to do it.

When your baby is about six months old it will not be the physical separation that will cause them anxiety (when they are out for the count they won't know you aren't watching their chest rise and fall like in those early days!). It is the re- sponse they get when they wake up and start crying or calling for you that matters; just like in the day, your baby will have their own language for night-time attention.

Sometimes you'll hear them, they'll grump for a few min- utes and go back to sleep without you having to lift your head from the pillow. Other times a quick cuddle for five to ten minutes will help them go back to sleep and you'll be able to return to your own bed. But then there are those nights when if they are not in your arms they will scream the place down. I don't know many mothers who haven't had nights like this. Some nights you'll have the energy to keep settling them back in their cot; other nights you and your partner will play musi- cal beds with one of you in the room with the baby and the other in the spare room or on the sofa just to get a few hours' shut-eye. There are no hard-and-fast rules here – do what you feel is best.

The important thing is that there is a big difference between grumping and a distressed baby that will cry and cry and cry. If your Little One is trying it on a bit, they'll soon fall asleep after five minutes or so. If they are feeling insecure, or are in pain, or hungry, then leaving them to cry all night is not going to make for a happy, well-attached baby in the long term. Some parents will tell you they left their baby to cry for a few nights and they soon learned to go through, and for me that's the crux of it – 'they *learned* not to cry'. To develop a lifelong bond with your child that is positive, well-balanced and nurturing, they need to learn that you are there for them. This doesn't mean you have to be around every single second, or that you can't go out or back to work. It does mean that someone, whether it is you, your partner or another caregiver, needs to be there to respond to your Little One when they need it. It doesn't have to be you that always gets up in the night, and like I said, some nights it's really not necessary, but when they need comfort, or pain relief, or fluids, it is really important their needs are met physically and emotionally. Security builds up gradually from the first few days and weeks after birth and during the early years. Following your own heart and feelings will almost always be right for you and your baby.

If you are having frequent or constant disturbed nights, then taking a look at your baby's general routine and feeding and napping patterns could help you all to get a better night's sleep. Have a look in Chapter 3 for some ideas for little things you might be able to tweak in your Little One's day.

Five Tips to Positively Help Your Baby's Development

This will not only help your baby's development but regular happy activity with you only increases their feelings of love and security.

1 **Tummy Time**
Right from the start give your baby opportunities for supervised Tummy Time every day (just start with five minutes and build up gradually).

2 **Fun every day**
Singing and playing with your baby every day makes the world of difference. It may only last a few minutes at a time in the midst of everyday tasks but it will make your baby happy and enhance their development.

3 **Baby talk**
Narrate what you are doing, have one-sided chats and leave a little gap for your baby to talk back – they'll soon be joining in with the conversation.

4 **Fresh air and exercise**
Lots of opportunities to get out and about in the fresh air helps both of you get what you need to be happy.

5 **Celebrate**
They may be only small, but enjoy and take pride in all your baby's achievements and fun together. It's the little things that really matter when it comes to happiness.

Being emotionally secure helps us know we are worthy of love

Feeling worthy of love and being loved is a starting point for the development of good mental health, self-confidence and high self-esteem. How you treat your child from their first days and the rest of their lives shapes their sense of self. A well-attached child is more likely to reciprocate with others and have positive relationships not only with family and friends but within the wider community and beyond. The people we grow into is rooted in those early years, when we are developing our feelings and understanding of ourselves and our place in the word.

3. Praise and recognition

It is funny that in the past proud parents rarely praised their baby (though I think this is no longer the norm today). In some families it might be because there's a belief that praise will spoil a child or make them 'big-headed'. Praise, though, is a vitally important part of your baby's emotional development. Not only will praise and encouragement help them develop stronger self-confidence and self-awareness, it tells your Little One that they are worthy of your love. This sense of self-worth will give your child a more positive image of themselves, which if it is continued throughout their childhood will stay with them for the whole of their lives and determine how they form relationships with others.

Praising your child when they do something new or to reinforce their developing skills, like feeding themselves or cruising along the sofa, will *not* make your child into a little emperor or a little tyrant; in fact, it will have the opposite effect, as children who do not receive positive praise and attention will often behave badly in order to try and stimulate attention from their parents.

Praising your child from an early age shows you love them

Knowing you are worthy of love is very different from the realisation that our parents love us. I have

often heard people say to an older child who is lacking praise and recognition from a parent, 'They love you in their own way, they just don't show it.' When this happens, whatever age the child is, they will not be aware they are loved if they are not shown it, so telling them in this way makes very little difference.

A parent is the most important person in a child's life. Knowing our parents believe in us is essential to our emotional well-being. Your baby can experience a sense of accomplishment and joy when you praise them. You are the centre of their world, and how you respond to what they do really matters.

At six months or so you may notice your Little One holds their back straight when sitting, though they may topple over. Encouraging them and giving them opportunities to practise this new skill surrounded by cushions and soft toys for a short time of supervised play every day doesn't just help their physical development but reinforces your love for them and gives them the happy feeling we all get when we are praised for doing something. We are all more likely to try something new when we feel safe and happy, and it's an opportunity for you to try something new, too – maybe it is baby yoga and seeing your flexible Little One get their foot to their mouth! Celebrating those moments when your baby starts to take their weight on their feet and stands or does a full press-up during Tummy Time are what make parenting so worthwhile and are all part of having a happy baby and being a happy family.

Being positive with your Little One helps them be a happy baby

Some parents (especially dads, I'm afraid) feel that you have to toughen children up with teasing and ridiculing. You cannot toughen up a child, let alone a baby, by pushing them into situations where they are frightened or unhappy. If children hear harsh and cajoling words it can create a mental freeze, and often they will grow into rigid and stubborn children, or they sometimes become frightened and extremely introverted. This doesn't mean you can't have fun with your baby; dads are often brilliant at getting their Little One to laugh and have lovely fun and games, but there is a difference between this and having a laugh at your child's expense.

I believe that from the moment of birth babies have an emotional need to hear praising words and to be treated with love and respect as an equal and individual human being. It is not probably something one consciously thinks about, more of an attitude, really, but once this seed is planted, positive parenting begins straight away in how you behave towards your baby, because our children's behaviour is affected by our own.

If positive parenting feels right for you, most likely you won't even have to think about it. Many parents can't stop themselves telling their Little One (and everyone else) how fantastic they are all the time – and thinking your baby is the best person on the planet and being thrilled with every little move they make. That is exactly the way it should be – your baby is very lucky to have you!

All babies deserve and need the same level of respect you would show for any other human being – they are a separate person in their own right, only ever so small, which means they probably need even more kind words and gentle praise and encouragement (I know I don't like it when people are harsh with me!). Acknowledging their achievements with praise and a cheerful word really works wonders. We all love to feel we've done something well and that we are recognised for it, and a baby is no different – in fact, they really crave positive attention from you.

Trust your baby to go at their own pace

As human beings we all need to strive to achieve, and there is no one like a baby for adopting the mantra 'Try, try, try again' – endeavour is their middle name! Your Little One will learn by their mistakes and they are entitled to fail, and need to know that this is acceptable to you. Just let them go at their own pace, and celebrate those small achievements because they are really rather wonderful, even if the only person who sees that is you.

Babies all develop at their own pace and as a parent all you can do is provide the opportunity to develop, like doing Tummy Time, singing, reading to them – but you can't make it happen. It's not helpful when people compare your baby to another – try and keep in mind that developmental milestones are just a rough guide, and every child is different. Some babies talk early, some walk early – when they do this is no reflection on you as a parent. If, however, you do feel worried about your baby's development, do talk to your doctor or a health professional. Nearly all parents worry, but there is a big difference between that and having a feeling that your baby may need treatment or extra support. It is your job to look out for your Little One, and it is the job of health professionals like me to support you. I've learned over the years that a mother's instinct is very powerful, and you should always listen to parents who are mostly with their baby every day, because they know them better than anyone.

It is good to notice as your baby progresses to a new development stage like being able to transfer objects from one hand to another or beginning to hand-feed at around eight months or so, but babies tend to do things in their own time and every baby is different. It is lovely in the time coming up to their first birthday when your Little One can sit playing completely absorbed in something for ten minutes or so before losing their balance, or toddling off to discover something new as they pull to stand and cruise along the edges of the furniture. Nearly all parents feel like the time just whizzes past, so enjoying those special moments is really worthwhile.

Enjoying your little one's achievements makes parenting a joy

Every day your baby will do something that makes you proud – and praise can also come in the form of a loving touch or a big cuddle; it doesn't always have to be rapturous applause. You don't have to be over the top or fake it, just respond naturally and show you are pleased and happy with what your baby is doing. A simple little phrase like 'Well done' or a smile will give your baby pleasure, and plenty of praise will only add to their sense of love and security.

4. New experiences

New experiences make up a vital part of your Little One's emotional and general development – helping to stimulate their thirst for knowledge and their understanding of themselves and the world around them. Everything is new to your baby, and it is wonderful to see the world through their eyes and the delight they take from the everyday things we take for granted. Play is a great way for developing interests with your baby. They will become curious about their world and how things work. Babies have a strong desire to explore. They love toys with a texture that is soft, and fuzzy material that makes a crinkly, crunchy or squeaky noise. It is mainly through play that children under five learn and develop new skills.

Sometimes playing with children comes naturally to parents, as many mums and dads find it so enjoyable. If your own parents didn't play with you it might take more effort to find ways for you to play with your baby. Even though play seems an obvious part of your baby's life, sometimes in the midst of feeding, baby care and tiredness, play starts to come a bit low down the priority list – but play doesn't just benefit your baby, it does you good, too. There will always be chores to do, so taking a little time every day to have some fun is just what is needed for happy babies and parents.

New experiences are something that can be big or small, planned or spontaneous and fun for all the family. It might sometimes be an experience like going to the park or library,

a group activity or a café where your baby will be in new surroundings, meeting new people and having new things to play with, getting lots of exercise and fun. But it can also be the small things like showing your baby the flowers in the garden in springtime, pulling laundry out of the basket when you are doing the washing, letting them see themselves in the mirror with you, or discovering their favourite song on the kitchen radio.

New experiences for your baby can give you precious time to get things done

When I picture a baby having a new experience I often think of my grandfather when he heard my baby brother cry. He'd take him to the window and say, 'What can we see? There's the postman bringing the letters and parcels. You can post a letter in a big red box; it's called a post box. Look at the green trees, see their leaves blowing in the wind?' He was simply describing the world around him. This just came naturally to him and I believe he would have scoffed if he had been told that this was a vital emotional need of all babies. It was something he just worked out for himself that helped make a baby happy and distracted them, giving my busy mother the chance to get things done.

When you do need to get things done, new experiences can be very helpful. It is my belief that a few well-chosen programmes on quality children's television will do your Little One no harm at all. You can watch together, and once they are settled take a moment to see to a task. I've often seen children do their first wave to a well-loved TV character, or

Talk to Your Baby Every Day

Even tiny babies benefit from you narrating your daily tasks to them and describing what you are doing. The sound of your voice is music to their ears, whether it's a story or an article from a magazine. Talking about the weather or what you are doing as you push your pram down the street is very interesting to your Little One.

dance along with the music. I'm not advocating putting your baby in front of the TV all day, but they do benefit from selective and limited television viewing which can stimulate learning and imagination and give you the chance to see to household tasks.

It's how you do it, not what you do, that counts

It is can be lovely to go on an outing with your Little One, but don't put too much pressure on yourself. Outings can be tiring and do require a bit of forethought and preparation on your part to be successful. So please don't feel you need to be organising Mary Poppins-like excursions every day, especially with a teething, grumpy baby where your best chance for a happy day may be to stay close to home.

You might experience pressure from other parents to go to classes and enrol your baby in costly activities. What you choose to do with your child is up to you; you don't have to commit to a weekly activity if it is more pressure than pleasure. Take a buffet approach: choose what you want and leave the rest. Your Little One will not be missing out; it is happy time spent with you that matters, and that can be anywhere. Groups where there are other positive parents and you enjoy socialising are great for you both – just do what makes you both happy.

It's *how* you spend time with your baby that really makes the difference. Like most things in parenting, it is having patience and a positive approach that can turn the mundane into a lovely new experience for both of you. No doubt you will have a natural ability to give your baby new experiences, and you'll most likely do this every day without even thinking about it, but it's nice to look over your activity with your Little

One sometimes and just note all the wonderful things you are doing to help them grow and develop. It may even be a good excuse for you to do something new, too.

5. Responsibility and discipline

Giving your child a sense of responsibility is an emotional need that is of greater and greater interest to parents as their child gets older. When it comes to babies, a 'good baby' does not mean they give their parents little or no trouble. In fact, 'good babies' are usually the result of a very hard-working parent who is working round the clock to make sure all their Little One's needs are met. They do get into a fair amount of trouble-making activity, but their parents expect it and don't punish them. Active children getting into cupboards and pulling everything off the bookcase is a part of their development. So if you want to keep inquisitive little fingers away from your precious things, then the simplest solution is to put them out of reach and use barriers and guards to prevent it happening.

As your child grows, giving them some choice and letting them have a little control can work wonders to prevent upset, and can be a useful distraction technique. As children grow they do often get into everything and it can be a frustrating time for many parents, but just how much can your baby understand about what they can and can't do?

Setting boundaries to keep your baby safe

When it comes to rule-making, keeping your child out of harm's way should be at the top of the list. Many of us grew up with rules about what children can and cannot do – often these are personal decisions, and what is important to one person doesn't matter to another.

As your Little One gets mobile, creating physical boundaries becomes more important. Your Little One is too young to understand the danger of stairs, knives in the kitchen drawer or the cooker. You can explain to them kindly and calmly why you can't let them in the cupboard under the kitchen sink, but don't expect them to take it in.

If your baby is getting into a situation that is dangerous or destructive, like putting their fingers in the electric socket or peeling the wallpaper off the walls, then verbal commands really don't work. You can say 'No' if you want to, but someone needs to get in there quickly, remove them from harm's way and give them something else to do instead. From six months you may notice your baby giving you a cheeky smile just as they are about to do something they shouldn't, but at this stage knowing doesn't translate into stopping, and you're a long way off from your Little One being able to have a sense of right and wrong, so no punishment or chastisement is needed as part of discipline and setting boundaries at this stage.

The difference between responsibility and discipline

Introducing the beginnings of responsibility and discipline with your baby is not easy, and at times very inconvenient. Punishment will not serve any purpose with a baby, as it will not act as a deterrent from them doing it again and is therefore *not* a part of positive parenting.

Being the decision-makers about what a child can and cannot do is the parents' responsibility, and it can be very draining when you can't use verbal commands yet and they are becoming very physically active. Many mums have told me they've felt they'd slipped into the role of disciplinarian and are making all the decisions, not just about what's a 'No-no' but about what the baby eats, sleeping patterns and techniques, choosing childcare and doing all the baby-proofing whilst Daddy gets to do all the 'fun stuff'. Parenthood, if you are in a relationship, is a partnership, and not only is it a good idea early on to reach agreement on your approach to positive parenting, but also not to put all the pressure of teaching self-discipline and retrieving your mischief-making Little One onto one parent. It's good for the whole family if you do take turns.

Don't let people label your child

All babies have their off moments and all babies will protest at something, whether that's getting dressed or having their hair washed. Just be aware of any well-meaning friends and family who start to label your child. Without meaning it people will start to refer to babies as 'the clever one' or 'the pretty one' or 'the naughty one', especially when there is more than one child in the family.

Not only can these become self-fulfilling prophecies if repeated too often, but they can be detrimental to a child's self-esteem. What all children need is positive attention – what the people around them say and do really does matter. Having a consistent and positive approach to setting boundaries, and praising them when they make progress, all help to make your Little One happy, feel loved and secure as well as keeping them safe and sound.

Let your little one make a few decisions

Giving your Little One some decision-making power is important, too. Babies will have a preference for what they want to eat first off their plate, or which toys they want to play with (though do ensure they only play with age-appropriate, safety-approved toys). These preferences are very small and barely discernible in everyday life, and no fanfare is required when they make their decisions, but it is nice to recognise you are giving your baby the opportunity to choose for themselves.

Putting food they can hand-feed themselves or a sippy cup on the tray of their high chair from when they are seven months or so gives your baby the opportunity to develop without pressure or expectation. Choice is important because if a child has no say over the things that happen to them they are more than likely going to become frustrated over those everyday tasks. It is normal for all children, including babies and toddlers, to protest loudly and fiercely when they have to do something they don't like – and poor Mummy! You wish you didn't have to wipe their face umpteen times a day, change their clothes and nappies all the time, especially when you get a very cross response from your Little One. Please resist the temptation to let negative words slip out, as it undoes all the positive parenting you are working so hard on. Having said that, everyone has the odd cross moment, so don't be too hard on yourself about it. Just apologise without too much fuss; it'll help show your Little One the way when they become toddlers and do start to learn about right and wrong. Everyone makes mistakes, and if we are sorry, the people we love forgive us and forget about it.

It's our old friends patience and perseverance again that are needed. All you can do is recognise your baby's discomfort and do your best to minimise it with soothing words and a few distractions to get it all over with as quickly as possible. Treating your baby with respect whilst doing the everyday things we all need to do, such as brushing our teeth, is all part of life and your child will come to realise this.

Growth and development ages and stages

The charts on the following pages demonstrate just a few things your baby might do at various ages – but there are many more, and the timings do vary. Have a little look for ideas of the fun experiences you can enjoy with your baby.

	0–3 months	3–6 months
Ready steady go	Grasping your finger and holding on tight	Holding head up well now
	Starting to do push-ups (i.e. lifts head when on tummy during supervised Tummy Time)	Starting to do real press-ups during Tummy Time
		Starting to hold objects, e.g. rattle, before throwing them
		During Tummy Time is getting more mobile, e.g. rolling, spinning and doing a dry 'swimming' motion
		Towards six months baby might sit momentarily before wobbling over

6-9 months	9-12 months
Sits momentarily and develops sitting more securely with practice	Starting to be mobile now. Crawling, and some babies walk with a push-along toy or even unaided
Many babies are rolling over and often can do both ways, but some babies rarely or never roll	Sitting very reliably, playing with toys on the floor
May be starting to crawl, bottom shuffle or both	Can get around the house by themselves
Likes to take their weight and stand, and may start to cruise around the furniture (avoid baby walkers as they are unsafe and may delay motor development)	

	0–3 months	3–6 months
Look and see	Starting to smile, which develops into a convincing, recognisable smile Gazing at you and looking towards light Staring at objects like curtains and blinds	Really smiling and getting excited by people and objects Animated and enthusiastic at the sight of food
Listen and learn	Stills to your voice and recognises it May like music and enjoys your singing	Vocalising more now with coos and gurgles Enjoys making lots of noise and will enjoy and recognise music and singing (babies can be soothed by music – anything from Mozart to rap

6-9 months	9-12 months
Starting to pick up little threads and bits using a pincer movement	Likes stories and looking in books and at pictures
Picking up food from baby tray and hand-feeding	May be starting to point with index finger
Play clapping games, e.g. Patty Cake. Enjoying favourite TV programmes, songs and books	Starting to drink water from baby cup and getting very proficient at hand-feeding
Vocalising now, starting with multiple syllables, e.g. Goo, goo, goo and Ga, ga, ga	Singing rhymes and playing 'Incy Wincey Spider' and 'Twinkle, Twinkle Little Star'
Laughing and squealing in response to things	May like going to groups like Bounce and Rhyme and Mums and Toddlers
	Understanding what is being said now and may be responding with single words

7

Keep It Simple – Wean Your Way

Weaning begins when your baby starts to have some solid food as well as breast or formula milk. In the beginning most of their nutrition will still come from their milk, but eventually they'll get everything they need from a diet of nutritionally well-balanced family foods. By the end of the first year a baby should be having three meals, one to two healthy snacks and a pint of milk a day.

Weaning can be fun – messy, but fun. You and your baby can get the most out of the experience by keeping it simple and following your Little One's lead. If you can use fresh foods most of the time, you'll be giving your baby a great introduction to food – but don't worry if some days it's easier to use quality ready-made baby food. Each baby has their own way of doing things; they might hand-feed at one meal and then demand to be spoon-fed at the next. Going with the flow and trying not to put high expectations on yourself and your baby is my approach for a happy baby and family.

When should I start to wean my baby?

Most babies are happy with only breast milk or formula milk for five months or so, and can stay feeding exclusively on milk until up to six months of age. You are the best judge of when your baby is ready to try a bit of solid food for the first time, and sometimes a few babies do start to wean as early as 18 weeks.

When your baby starts to wean it is fine to give them encouragement and show how much you are enjoying this experience together, but try and resist the urge to go over the top. Giving your Little One excessive praise for doing something like eating, which after all is a part of everyday life, sets a precedent. A smile and saying 'Well done' is enough to recognise and encourage them without making too much of a song and dance about it. Giving them a little choice about what to eat and the opportunity to sample some finger foods whilst you spoon-feed or pop some food into their mouths will help your Little One take baby steps towards taking responsibility for hand-feeding.

All this takes time and it is unrealistic to expect babies to exclusively hand-feed because, until they are seven to eight months old, most babies do not have the control or the pincer grip needed to hold food well enough to eat completely unaided. A balance between giving them opportunities to explore the textures of finger foods, combined with spoon-feeding to ensure they get their nutritional needs met, will provide the practical and emotional support your Little One needs during weaning. You want it to be a positive experience for both of you, and there will be days when they refuse everything, spit out their food and chuck the meal you've lovingly prepared onto the floor. This can be very disheartening, but in the early days of weaning it is the experience that matters. It's not that you've done anything wrong, it's simply your baby doing what babies do.

Giving your baby their first foods

You've noticed the signs your baby is ready to taste their first solid foods, which is quite exciting. Follow these simple steps to make up their first meal. Tea-time is a good time of day to start, but pick a time that is right for your family.

If your Little One spits out the food or shows little interest, leave it another one to two weeks before you try again. If your baby is enjoying their first tastes, try again at the same time the next day. Gradually introduce different foods, but don't overwhelm them with too many tastes all at once. If your Little One eats all their food very quickly and is looking for more, double the quantity at their next meal to 4 teaspoons; see whether they finish it or whether it's a bit too much. Use your own judgement about what feels right for your baby. Whatever you try, it'll just be little amounts to start with as your baby's stomach is only the size of their clenched fist. When they've had enough they've had enough, so there's no need to push.

Most mums start with milder yellow and orange vegetables like carrots or butternut squash. Try to introduce only a couple of new tastes a week to start with, to give your baby the opportunity to discover each flavour. Be prepared that your Little One won't like every taste and there will some spitting out, pulling faces and showing their disgust for certain flavours. This can be a little upsetting when you've lovingly made up a batch of purée. It's all about discovery, so if they don't like something, freeze the rest of the batch and try it again a month or so later.

Happy Baby Five Weaning Signs

1 **I'm not happy**

Have you noticed that your LO isn't as content lately?
Are they demanding the next feed earlier and earlier?
Have they started to wake in the night for a feed when
they were previously sleeping through?

2 **Give me some**

Every time you or the people around you are eating,
is your baby watching intently? Does your LO put their
fist in their mouth and get all vocal when mealtimes
come around? (Some babies do show curiosity when
you eat from an early stage, so doing only this wouldn't
indicate they are ready to wean; it is when this is
combined with other signs.)

3 **Little weight change**

Has your baby not gained weight recently or even had
a slight fall from their usual weight centile line? It may
be they need the extra nutrients from solid food. (If
you do have any concerns about weight, talk to your
health visitor or doctor.)

4 **Sitting up well**

Does your baby sit up well independently or with
support? This is important, because babies need to
be in an upright position to safely swallow solid food.
If your baby is not quite ready for the high chair, the
support of a rubber chair like a Bumbo will give them
the security and safety they need.

5 **Give me some more**

Did your baby smack their lips and want some more when you tried them with a little something? If you make up just a small bowl of baby rice with some breast or formula milk and they yum it up, they are ready to wean. If they aren't really interested but are showing the other signs, leave it a week or two before you try again.

How to Make Your Baby's First Meal

1 Sterilise the bowl and weaning spoon (if they are under six months).

2 Put 2 teaspoons of plain baby rice into a bowl.

3 Mix in 2 teaspoons of expressed breast milk or warmed formula milk and stir with a weaning spoon until it is a smooth paste (you don't want it to be too solid or too runny, so you can always add a little more milk to make the right consistency).

You can also give your baby a little fruit or vegetable purée mixed with the prepared baby rice or on its own.

Vegetables
Avocado
Butternut squash
Carrots
Parsnips
Root vegetables

Fruit
Apples
Bananas
Pears
Plums

Cereals and Pulses
Baby rice
Porridge
Tiny orange lentils
(Dahl)
Sweet potato

If your baby is Caucasian and you start to notice their skin gets an orange glow, it may be from too many orange-coloured vegetables. Switch to another vegetable for a few days before giving them their favourite carrots or sweet potato again. Soft foods like ripe avocado or banana just need thorough mashing with a fork. Stay away from soft fruits like strawberries or raspberries until your baby is older, as they can cause very loose motions and give your baby explosive nappies. Also leave citrus fruits until your Little One is eight to ten months and hand-feeding. Choose seedless tangerine varieties and ensure any stone fruits like plums or nectarines have the stone removed right up until primary school age, as they are a choking hazard.

Trust Yourself

Sterilise Your Baby's Dinner Service

When babies first try solid foods, if they are under six months you'll need to sterilise their bowl and weaning spoon. Make sure you thoroughly hand-wash and rinse off all the soap residue before sterilising.

How to Purée

1 Chop up fruit or vegetables into small pieces.

2 Gently stew in a saucepan, using only a little freshly drawn water so it is not too wet when puréed.

3 Mash with a fork or push the cooked fruit or veg through a plastic sterilised sieve into a sterilised bowl (do not add anything to it like sugar, salt or honey).

Once your baby is well established in having baby rice you can move on to porridge and unsweetened breakfast cereals. Avoid wholewheat breakfast cereals and biscuits as they are very rough on the gut, and too much roughage makes for very sore bottoms. You can also try cooking a small quantity of the tiny orange lentils that break down and go mushy for 20 to 25 minutes or so before adding them to a vegetable purée when you feel your baby is ready for a bit more diversity in their diet.

Foods to Avoid During the First Year

It is recommended that you avoid giving your baby foods they might be allergic to. **Avoid:**

Soft and blue cheese
Cured meats, e.g. salami
Raw eggs
Honey
Whole nuts
Pâté

Salt
Shellfish
Smoked salmon
Sugar
Sweetener
Unpasteurised dairy
Wholewheat

Second tastes

When your baby reaches six months you can safely start to introduce more foods at mealtimes. Once your baby is polishing off their tea-time meal, start giving them breakfast after their first milk feed. Cereal with fruit, or baby rice with fruit, makes for a lovely, easy-to-prepare and nutritious first meal of the day. If you're looking for ideas on what to serve your Little One, there are sample

Trust Yourself

Your LO Still Needs Their Milk

Your baby will still need their milk feed as well as any meals or snacks. First foods provide a bit of extra sustenance, but it is the experience that counts. Your LO will still get the majority of their nutritional needs met through their milk.

meal plans at the end of this chapter. As a guide, breakfast may be 9–10 am and tea-time 4–5 pm, but choose the times that are right for your baby and your family. You don't have to follow a strict regime; if your baby is napping contentedly, that's fine, or if they show no interest in having lunch one day it's not a big deal – just watch for their cues when they later need a milk feed or some food.

Babies do tend to shudder a bit when they taste some foods. This is usually

due to the wetness of a purée, and there is nearly always some spitting out and playing with their food. You can expect hands to go in the bowl, that they'll grab the spoon off you and that at some stage your Little One will tip the contents of their meal over themselves, their high chair, the furniture and floor. This is not only normal but a very useful learning experience, and it is good they are enjoying mealtimes even though it may seem like it's for the wrong reasons.

Very few people like all tastes; a few new tastes a week is a great start to weaning, but when you discover their favourite food resist the temptation to give it them too often. Babies often suddenly reject the food they loved yesterday

Happy Baby Second Foods: from 6 Months

As well as all the first foods, once your baby is over six months they can start to enjoy:

Vegetables
Asparagus
Broccoli
Cauliflower
Celeriac
Cucumber
Green beans
Greens
Leeks
Peas
Swedes

Fruit
Apricot
Kiwi fruit
Mango
Melon
Nectarine
Peach

Pulses
Beans

Dairy
Cheddar cheese
(grated)
Fromage frais
Full-fat cows' milk in
cooking
Yoghurt

Protein
Chicken
Fish

Carbohydrate
Pasta
Rice

These are just a few suggestions; there are many, many more.

and refuse it for months; if this happens, just leave it a while before you serve it up again.

Home-freezing

Allow food to thoroughly cool down before home-freezing. Place into sterilised containers with a label on for the date it was frozen – and it's a good idea to write what it is, as mushed baby food all looks the same once it is an ice cube. You can keep baby food for about eight weeks in the freezer. When you remove it, allow it to fully thaw for several hours and then heat gently in a saucepan, checking the temperate is not too hot before you serve it to your Little One. Once you have defrosted a meal it cannot be frozen again. I wouldn't recommend using the microwave, as it can create hot spots that burn a baby's mouth.

Using shop-bought baby foods

There are lots of ready-made baby foods for sale. Making your own is cheaper and more nourishing, and does give your baby the opportunity to eat with the rest of the family. There is, though, nothing wrong with giving ready-made baby food. These foods are extremely convenient and can be really handy to have in if you are out and about, or if your baby is experiencing teething pain and won't chew their food properly;

Happy Baby Second Foods: 8–12 Months

Between eight months and a year you can start to introduce these foods as well into your LO's diet:

Vegetables
Cherry tomatoes (halved)
Courgettes
Tomatoes (cut up)

Fruit
Apricots
Blueberries (halved)
Clementines
Dried fruit
Grapes (halved)
Grapefruit
Raisins
Satsumas

Pulses
Baked beans

Dairy
Butter
Cheese triangles
Custard

Protein
Chickpeas
Eggs
Meat
Puy lentils

Carbohydrate
Breadsticks
Chapattis
Noodles
Pancakes
Pikelets
White pitta bread
Rice cakes
Risotto
White toast triangles

This is just a selection of foods to choose from.

a chilled weaning pouch might be just what they need to get their nutrients as easily and pain-free as possible so they don't rely on milk alone at this stage.

I'd recommend high-quality organic baby brands or freshly chilled ready-made foods, but the choice is yours. Nutritionally these can meet your baby's dietary needs, but it can make switching to family foods harder if they are exclusively fed on ready-made baby foods.

Vitamin supplements

Vitamin supplements can be a useful addition to your baby's diet, and come in lots of different forms. Ask your local pharmacist for a recommendation that is suitable to your baby's age and needs.

Moving on to hand-feeding and family foods

You don't have to specially prepare each meal for your baby. Keep it simple and use the fresh foods you are eating or cooking for yourself by blending and puréeing some for your Little One to enjoy. From seven to eight months some babies will be ready to have a lunchtime meal as well as breakfast and tea. Try giving them some lunch at midday if that works for you.

When your Little One can do the pincer grip and can hold objects between their thumb and finger, you can start to serve foods they can safely hand-feed as an accompaniment to their spoon-fed meals. Put a spoon on the tray of their high chair, some foods to hand-feed, and give them the opportunity to choose whether to pick up some of their own food, play with a spoon or be fed by you. It's quite usual for babies to mix it up.

Trust Yourself

Two Spoons at Mealtimes

If your baby wants to have a play with the spoon or even have a go at feeding themselves, use two spoons at mealtimes: one for you and one for them. That way you can feed your LO without having a fight on your hands.

Hand-feeding

Always stay with your child while they are eating and ensure they are strapped into a high chair; accidents happen in just a moment. When your baby starts to hand-feed it is a real high point in your weaning journey, but be careful of foods that could get stuck in the windpipe and choke your baby. Fruits and vegetables like cherry tomatoes, grapes and blueberries are just the right size to cause a blockage, so do take care and halve them before serving. Slice up a banana and break each wheel into three; peel an apple, take out the core and quarter; the peeled end of a cucumber is a great teether as well as a snack; and cutting a piece of white toast into four triangles prevents your baby from gagging on too big a piece or choking on a small piece.

Cooking for your family

Family foods like casserole or poached chicken are beautifully soft for homemade baby food and freeze well. When you're cooking the family meal, don't use stock cubes or salt (you can add salt to your portion when you serve it if you need to). Instead make a salt-free base by softly cooking onions, carrots and celery in a little oil or butter. Add in some water and sweat down gently for 15 minutes or so until very tender.

From six months you can introduce cows' milks in cooking and make your baby a rice pudding or a lovely white sauce. When cooking fish, take extra care the bones are removed; make friends with your local fishmonger and they will do it for you. A fillet of white fish in white sauce with a little mashed potato and vegetables is a well-balanced family meal.

Happy Baby Family Food Suggestions

Beef casserole	Poached chicken
Beef lasagne	Roast dinners
Chicken goujons	Salmon
Eggy bread and beans	Sandwich triangles
Fish fingers	Shepherd's pie
Fish pie	Homemade soup
Lamb hotpot	Spaghetti bolognese
Macaroni cheese	Stew
Pasta bake	White fish
Pikelets with toasted cheese	

Using a tippy or sippy cup and switching to cows' milk

From six months some babies are ready to start having a go with a tippy or sippy cup, or a smaller open cup if you prefer. Once your baby is having three meals a day and is confidently handling their food, pop a closed cup onto their tray. Don't comment on it being there or go over the top if they start to drink from it; just calmly see what happens. If they pay no attention to the cup at all, leave it for a few weeks before introducing it again.

There are lots of different beakers to choose from and I think the simpler the better, but the choice is yours. You can switch to giving your baby an easy-to-hold open cup once you think they are ready – but be prepared for some spills.

By your Little One's first birthday they will probably be ready for three meals, a milky supper and two little snacks. They still need a pint of milk a day, but that can be made up from the milk they have in cooking, dairy products as well as any remaining milk feeds. You can start to give your baby cold cows' milk in their cereal and as a drink if you want to. At this time many babies start to drop their milk feeds as their appetite increases. Follow your baby's lead – it's always a bit of trial and error, as their feeding pattern will shift throughout the early years.

Once they are drinking regularly from the cup, you can start to make a gradual switch over from using a bottle to the cup. Start with their morning drink, then tea-time, then lunchtime, snack time and eventually their night-time bottle. Don't worry too much if your baby still needs the comfort of the bottle for their night-time feed. Do what feels right for your baby – they will get there.

If you notice a sudden dip in your baby's appetite, it might be that they no longer need their morning milk feed. Try replacing their morning milk with another drink like cooled boiled water, or just a couple of teaspoons of natural apple or orange juice heavily diluted if you want to. Never give squash or sugar-free drinks. The sweeteners dry the mouth, making your baby constantly thirsty and causing them to fill up their tummies with fluids, which reduces their appetite. The artificial colours and additives in these drinks don't have a positive impact on children's behaviour, either. If their appetite doesn't improve, talk to your health visitor or doctor; it may be teething pain or feeling unwell that is putting them off their food, especially if they are more clingy than usual, easily upset and are displaying other signs of teething or illness like rubbing their gums, coughing, red cheeks and strong-smelling wee and slightly runny poos.

Trust Yourself

A Milky Supper to Help Your LO Sleep

Giving your baby a milky supper like cereal or porridge before bed or their last milk feed will help them get to sleep more easily and sleep through the night.

Meal plan suggestions

The meal planners on the following pages indicate the variety of meal choices you can pick from. When you begin weaning, start with small quantities for one meal a day. Gradually increase the portion size, steadily introducing new flavours and textures and building towards giving your baby two meals a day. Your baby will still need the same number of milk feeds when you start to wean, and you can still feed on demand. It is good to have a rough timetable in your head so you can plan your day and have everything you need to meet your baby's needs, but don't worry too much about having a strict routine; things will shift slightly every couple of weeks during weaning. Follow your baby's lead.

Happy Baby Meal Planner 5+ Months

Simple suggestions to pick and choose from

	Breakfast	Mid-morning	Lunch
Monday	Milk feed on waking Baby rice	Milk feed	Milk feed
Tuesday	Milk feed on waking Baby rice with apple purée	Milk feed	Milk feed
Wednesday	Milk feed on waking Baby rice with pear purée	Milk feed	Milk feed
Thursday	Milk feed on waking Baby rice with plum purée	Milk feed	Milk feed
Friday	Milk feed on waking Baby rice with mushed banana	Milk feed	Milk feed
Saturday	Milk feed on waking Baby porridge made with baby's milk and fruit purée	Milk feed	Milk feed
Sunday	Milk feed on waking Baby yoghurt with fruit purée and a piece of white toast cut into triangles	Milk feed	Milk feed

Visit www.sarahbeeson.org for Meal Planner templates and recipe ideas.

Mid-afternoon	Tea-time	Bedtime
Milk feed	Baby rice Milk feed	Milk feed
Milk feed	Baby rice with carrot purée Milk feed	Milk feed
Milk feed	Baby rice with parsnip purée Milk feed	Milk feed
Milk feed	Baby rice with butternut squash purée Milk feed	Milk feed
Milk feed	Baby rice with sweet potato purée Milk feed	Milk feed
Milk feed	Baby rice with mashed avocado Milk feed	Milk feed
Milk feed	Carrot purée and previously cooked and cooled orange lentils Milk feed	Milk feed

Happy Baby Meal Planner 7+ Months

Simple suggestions to pick and choose from

	Breakfast	Mid-morning
Monday	Milk feed on waking Baby porridge with banana mash or wheels on high-chair tray	Milk feed
Tuesday	Milk feed on waking Baby yoghurt served with mashed or small pieces of mango on high-chair tray, and cheese spread on a triangle of white toast	Milk feed
Wednesday	Milk feed on waking Baby cereal with fresh or dried apricots	Milk feed
Thursday	Milk feed on waking Fromage frais with textured peach or nectarine	Milk feed
Friday	Milk feed on waking Baby muesli with previously boiled and cooled cows' milk	Milk feed
Saturday	Milk feed on waking Baked beans with white toast triangles and a selection of fruit	Milk feed
Sunday	Milk feed on waking Porridge with grated apple or pear	Milk feed

Visit www.sarahbeeson.org for Meal Planner templates and recipe ideas.

Lunch	Mid-afternoon	Tea-time	Bedtime
Milk feed	Milk feed	Mashed butternut squash and little pasta shells with grated cheese	Milk feed
Milk feed	Milk feed	Mashed sweet potatoes with orange lentils	Milk feed
Milk feed	Milk feed	Mashed cauliflower cheese and mashed asparagus or avocado	Milk feed
Milk feed	Milk feed	Puréed poached chicken in a white sauce with pea purée	Milk feed
Milk feed	Milk feed	White fish (take crumbs off one cooked fish finger) with pea and mashed potato purée	Milk feed
Milk feed	Milk feed	Tuna or salmon with small pasta shells in a cheese or white sauce	Milk feed
Milk feed	Milk feed	Blended roast chicken dinner, vegetables and baby gravy	Milk feed

At around 9 months most babies will be developing their hand-feeding skills and will be ready for lunch, snacks and a milky supper. You may find that as their appetite increases they will demand fewer milk feeds.

Happy Baby Meal Planner 9+ Months

Simple suggestions to pick and choose from

	Breakfast	Mid-morning	Lunch
Monday	Rice Crispies with cows' milk Offer a cup of milk or water	6 grapes (halved) Milk or water	Tuna and mashed sweetcorn with mini-jacket potato Offer a cup of water
Tuesday	Brioche eggy bread with fruit Offer a cup of milk or water	Mini-yoghurt pot Milk or water	Vegetable soup with breadsticks Offer a cup of water
Wednesday	Cheerios with cows' milk and halved blueberries Offer a cup of milk or water	Raisins Milk or water	Cooked lentils with sweet potato Offer a cup of water

Visit www.sarahbeeson.org for Meal Planner templates and recipe ideas.

Mid-afternoon	Tea-time	Bedtime
End of cucumber\n\nMilk or water	Chicken casserole with vegetables\n\nOffer a cup of water	Instant porridge or breakfast cereal with warmed cows' milk and/or buttered white toast\n\nMilk feed
¼ packet of carrot puffs\n\nMilk or water	Shepherd's pie with sweet potato mash\n\nOffer a cup of water	Instant porridge or breakfast cereal with warmed cows' milk and/or buttered white toast\n\nMilk feed
Half a banana\n\nMilk or water	Lamb hotpot\n\nOffer a cup of water	Instant porridge or breakfast cereal with warmed cows' milk and/or buttered white toast\n\nMilk feed

Happy Baby Meal Planner 9+ Months

Simple suggestions to pick and choose from

	Breakfast	Mid-morning	Lunch
Thursday	Scrambled egg with white toast triangles Offer a cup of milk or water	Baby biscuit and fruit Milk or water	Sandwiches (white bread) and raw red pepper and carrot pieces Offer a cup of water
Friday	Breakfast cereal with fruit Offer a cup of milk or water	Apple pieces Milk or water	Ham and cheese pancakes Offer a cup of water
Saturday	Boiled egg and white toast triangles Offer a cup of milk or water	Satsuma Milk or water	Homemade cheese and tomato pizza slices with cucumber and tomatoes Offer a cup of water
Sunday	Pancakes with yoghurt and apple or blueberry Offer a cup of milk or water	Chopped avocado Milk or water	Roast chicken dinner Offer a cup of water

Visit www.sarahbeeson.org for Meal Planner templates and recipe ideas.

Mid-afternoon	Tea-time	Bedtime
2 broccoli trees Milk or water	Macaroni cheese with tomatoes Offer a cup of water	Instant porridge or breakfast cereal with warmed cows' milk and/or buttered white toast Milk feed
Halved cherry tomatoes Milk or water	Fish pie with broccoli Offer a cup of water	Instant porridge or breakfast cereal with warmed cows' milk and/or buttered white toast Milk feed
Chopped or sliced melon Milk or water	Stir-fried vegetables and noodles Offer a cup of water	Instant porridge or breakfast cereal with warmed cows' milk and/or buttered white toast Milk feed
Half a pear Milk or water	Pikelets with toasted cheese Offer a cup of water	Instant porridge or breakfast cereal with warmed cows' milk and/or buttered white toast Milk feed

8

Teething and Caring for Your Baby's Teeth

Babies can have teeth at birth, although this is rare, and a few babies' teeth do come through in the first few months. Generally a baby's first teeth can appear anywhere from three months to past a year. You may notice the signs of teething weeks before even the tiniest tip of a tooth makes an appearance. Your Little One has 20 teeth to pop through, with the last four molars finally coming through usually around their second birthday. Some teeth will pop through with no trouble at all, and others will seem to take forever. There are many remedies for helping your baby through teething, but the biggest comfort of all will be sympathy and cuddles from you.

All your baby's milk teeth are already in place below the surface of the gum at birth. These start to move and work their way up slowly, often from two to three months. It's a constant stopping and starting process, which is why you can have a perfectly happy baby one day and a very grumpy one the next. There is no set pattern to teething; teeth can come through at any time and in any order. A lot of babies do get the bottom front two teeth first followed by the top two teeth at four to six months. Others start with side teeth and get the canines first, and a rare few their back teeth first. A few Little Ones don't get their first tooth until after their first birthday.

Your Baby's Teeth

Bottom front teeth (incisors)
Top front teeth (incisors)
Top lateral incisors (either side of the top front teeth)
Bottom lateral incisors (either side of the bottom front teeth)
Canines (sides of the mouth)
Premolars (behind the canines)
Molars (back teeth)

The 10 signs of teething

You'll know your Little One is teething if they are excessively dribbling, putting their fist in their mouth, or have red cheeks and tender gums. It may be a while before your Little One's teeth pop through, but you'll know something is going on when they just don't seem their usual happy selves. You may not see all these signs or even any of them; every baby is different when it comes to teething.

1. Trouble feeding

When your baby starts to teethe (which can happen at any time) you may notice they have trouble feeding. This is because they are hungry and want to feed but keep rejecting the breast or the bottle because their gums hurt and the nipple or teat is making them even sorer. Even if they start to feed they can break off to have a bit of a cry and a moan about their sore gums.

2. Dribbling

Lots of dribble, damp clothes, a wet bib or top are all signs your baby's imminent teeth are making them a bit drooly. You may notice your baby gets a teething rash or sore patches on their cheeks, chin, neck or chest. As your baby gets older and learns to swallow excess saliva you may notice they get loose motions as a result of all that extra fluid.

3. Grumpiness, crying and distress

If your baby is out of sorts and crying much more than usual, check to see if they've got any other signs of teething. Their bad day might be due to very sore gums. Check the signs of colic in the A–Z section to figure out whether it is pain in their tummy or their teeth and gums that is making them upset (often it is unfortunately a combination of both). If your baby has a raised temperature, get them checked over by your doctor.

4. Red cheeks

Reddening and sore-looking cheeks with a higher colour than usual may mean your baby is feeling the ill-effects of teething. You might notice them rubbing their rosy red cheeks too and looking very sorry for themselves.

5. Biting and gnawing

You might find your baby will suddenly give you a nip, or starts using random objects to massage their sore gums.

6. Teething cough and runny nose

A tickly cough accompanied by a runny nose that doesn't develop into a cold is a teething symptom from milk teeth to wisdom teeth.

7. 'Ammonia wee' and alkaline spot burns on bottom

From eight months or so you may notice the wee in your baby's nappy smells very strong, and they may have tiny burns from the alkaline urine that look like tiny rash-like dots. Keep them well hydrated and put a protective greasy coating of bottom butter or petroleum jelly on their bottoms to provide a barrier to prevent the wee touching the skin. If they do get sore, use nappy rash cream until it heals, then switch to using a greasy layer until they no longer have ammonia wee.

8. Waking up in the night

If your baby starts to wake up in the night in distress it may be the movement in their gums is causing them discomfort and pain. If you find they are waking for another milk feed, it could be that they need more milk or food during the day to help them sleep through. Look back on your day at their feeding and sleeping patterns and note how much they've eaten or whether they slept too long during their daytime nap. If you think they are in pain rather than hungry, give them pain relief first to see if they'll go back to sleep without a top-up feed, as waking up for a midnight snack might become a habit that's hard to break.

9. Ear-pulling, shaking and banging their heads

If you notice your baby pulling their ears and shaking or banging their head it may be they are trying to relieve the pain caused by their aching gums. Yanking their ears could also be caused by an ear infection, however, so if you're worried do talk to your health visitor or doctor.

10. Bumpy or hard gums

When you look in your baby's mouth you might notice red and angry gums that are hot to the touch. Or they may be a bit lumpy and bumpy, or very hard where the teeth are getting ready to push through the surface of the gum.

How to help your teething baby

Once your baby is over three months old you'll be able to go to the pharmacy and talk about the different teething remedies you can use to make life a little easier for your teething babe. Never give more than one teething or pain-relief product at the same time. They often have similar ingredients that shouldn't be used together. Paracetamol products and ibuprofen products shouldn't be given without medical supervision until your Little One is over six months old.

How to apply teething remedies (gels, powders and liquids)

If your baby is having problems feeding, try rubbing either teething gel, powder or liquid over their gums with a clean, dry finger before you start a feed, to help numb their gums a little so they can feed better. Babies often don't co-operate when you are trying to rub their gums, and it can be frustrating for you as they put up their little fists and knock your hand away when you're only trying to help them.

When your baby is calm, try facing them forwards on your lap and applying the teething remedy from behind, bringing your hand from underneath their chin so they won't see you coming.

You may also want to use baby paracetamol (if your baby is old enough) as well as a specific teething product if they seem to be having a really bad day.

Rubbing with an electric toothbrush

You can massage your baby's gums with the wet head of a little battery-operated baby toothbrush for a few seconds to see if it relieves the pain a bit.

Keep their fluids up

Teething babies need to be kept well hydrated. Regularly offer them a drink of water as well as their usual milk feed.

Pain relief

From six months you can give medication such as paracetamol oral suspension or ibuprofen products. If your baby starts teething before six months, discuss with your doctor whether it would be appropriate to give them pain-relief medications.

Teethers

There are many types of teethers and teething rings on the market. You may find your baby likes to use these to relieve their sore gums. If your Little One is under six months, sterilise the teethers and always clean them regularly. Always supervise your baby whilst they are using any teether. Avoid amber beads teething necklaces. They pose both a choking and a strangulation hazard.

Cold

You can use a frozen teething ring (under constant supervision). An icy cold teether works by relieving the gums through both massage and cooling. Do not use ice cubes or ice lollies as they are a choking risk.

Raise their mattress

If they have a teething cough or cold, try raising the head end of their mattress by putting a pillow or folded blanket or muslin underneath the mattress (you cannot use a pillow for a baby under a year old). Having their head and chest elevated will help reduce the trickle-back of saliva and mucus that hits the back of the throat and makes them cough.

Sympathy

You may find your baby cries more than usual, is wakeful and harder to calm, and needs lots of extra cuddles and reassurance. Babies love sympathy (don't we all?), so just make those soothing noises so they know Mummy and Daddy understand. The waves of pain a baby experiences don't usually last long, but your baby won't know it will all be over soon.

Use one of the calming techniques that usually work to soothe your baby. Teething often occurs alongside the development of attachment, which can result in very clingy Little Ones. Swiftly attending to their needs and staying calm helps to relieve their teething symptoms as soon as possible. Trust yourself: you know what will make your baby happy. Having a few distraction techniques to get you both through the day will often be called for. So a nice toy, a yummy snack, singing, reading a story or a little TV may all help get your Little One back on track to being a happy baby.

Teething and breastfeeding

Breastfeeding can be a huge comfort to a teething baby, giving them the extra fluids and the contact they need when nothing else will do. You'll find lots of patience and perseverance are needed when teething makes your baby fractious during breastfeeding. Remember what you did to calm you both in those early days of breastfeeding. Most mums will find it difficult and frustrating to try and feed a cross and hungry baby, but you will get through it; when new teeth are coming through the situation usually only lasts for a few days at a time.

Teething can present new challenges for breastfeeding mums. You may find that as soon as they start to feed they come off the breast crying with sore gums. It is important to try and give them some relief before you continue with the feed, or life is going to be very difficult and upsetting for you both.

Some mums find a baby with hard gums makes their nipples sore, so do use a nipple gel for yourself as well as a teething gel for them. If feeding your baby is causing you pain and discomfort even after applying teething remedies, then take your baby off the breast by breaking the seal with your little finger, then take a few moments and some deep breaths. Your baby may be using your nipple as a teether, and that is not something most women would want to endure for long (your baby has plenty of other options for rubbing those gums).

You could try using a nipple shield, or introducing some expressed breast milk for a while to give your nipples a break. What you don't want to happen is to let your nipples get very sore; if they do, you need to give them time to heal. You'll find the right solution that works for you – it's all trial and error and no fault of yours at all. If biting does become a habit you can't get your baby to break and it is causing you difficulty, now may be the time to start to think about gradually moving from breastfeeding to a bottle. It is well worth keeping on breastfeeding as long as you want to, but don't feel guilty if you feel you want to make a change. Trust your instincts: you'll know if this is a temporary situation that will be over when that tooth finally comes through.

It can be really helpful to talk to other mums or ask for extra support from health professionals or breastfeeding counsellors. It might just be that you need to share the frustration for a few days to get you through it. You can never predict how teething is going to work out; some babies teeth for ages but don't get any teeth until well after their first birthday, and others are born with teeth. For a few mums, teething goes smoothly, maybe they only have a few difficult days; other mums have a baby who seems to be teething all the time. You have no control over this, and we can't predict when and for how long a baby will teethe. Just do what feels right for you and your baby.

Teething and bottle-feeding

When your Little One is teething, take the opportunity to give them lots of extra cuddles, kisses and soothing words – they'll love a bit of sympathy and it'll help distract them from those waves of teething pain. Just check as well that you are using the right size teat, as there's a chance your baby is getting all frustrated because the flow of formula milk isn't right for them, especially if you haven't noticed any teething signs.

I know it makes you feel awful when they spit out the bottle and give you those reproachful looks, and then they start crying with hunger to make matters worse. This is no fault of yours, and all you can do is stay calm and try and soothe them and give them some teething remedies. It's not you; it's their sore gums that are making them cry.

Looking after your baby's teeth

As soon as your baby gets their first pearly whites you can start to gently brush their teeth with a wet baby toothbrush and with a tiny amount of baby toothpaste if you want to. If your Little One is still only two to three months old, just use water, as there is no need for toothpaste yet. Even if you just brush for a few seconds, the aim is to get your baby used to brushing their teeth twice a day as part of their daily routine.

Avoid sugary foods and drinks, as delaying giving your baby sugar will help to prevent tooth decay from their earliest days. Change your baby's toothbrush at least every three months as bacteria builds up on them and the bristles become hard and rough around the edges.

When your baby can brush their own teeth, let them have a go under careful supervision. Join in or follow up by giving them a more thorough clean yourself with a second toothbrush.

9

Leaving Your Baby in Someone Else's Care and Going Back to Work

During your first year with your baby it is quite likely that at some point you will need to leave them. It might be occasionally or regularly, to go out for a few hours or to return to full-time or part-time work. There is no right time to leave your baby and it is different from family to family depending on their circumstances. What is important is that you feel confident that whoever will be caring for your Little One while you are away will be able to meet their practical and emotional needs.

If you are going back to work, many parents find this a challenging experience. Even if you decide to be at home with your baby there will probably be times when you need to leave them with someone else. So it is useful to think about what childcare support is a good fit for your family and what you can do to prepare you and your baby for the separation. Many mums do worry about returning to work all through their maternity leave. It's natural to want to plan and have everything figured out, but don't let the anxiety spoil the precious time you have with your baby. Pre-planning, thinking ahead and trying things out are helpful, but it is your ability to respond positively to change that is an essential skill in parenting, and life with a baby changes continuously – that will go on past their first year and it is impossible to plan for everything. Your focus needs be on your baby, yourself and your family, and doing what is right for you.

Build up to leaving your baby gradually

When your baby experiences separation from you for long periods of time, especially if it is frequent, this can be a source of insecurity for both of you. This doesn't mean that a good parent cannot leave their baby; of course there may be occasions when you need to be away. What may cause insecurity is a sudden change. As long as there is a very responsive and good alternative carer for your baby, leaving your baby for a few hours will not cause them any harm, and if you can it will be better for everyone if you build up the length of time you are away gradually. It can also be a really good opportunity for your partner to get more involved and build a stronger relationship with your Little One and give you a much-needed break. Or if a grandparent or someone else is taking the role of the main carer while you are away, as long as they meet your baby's needs and make them feel loved and secure, this is a good option, too. It is important for your baby to have you near, but they'll need to get used to other people as well.

If you're breastfeeding you'll need to express some milk and freeze it so there's a good supply for the times you'll be away. Have a chat with the carer about the normal shape of your Little One's day, so they know roughly when they need to feed or what is their favourite song or which is their favourite toy; all those little things that are familiar and help to make your baby feel secure.

Leaving Your Baby for the First Time

If you are going to be away for more than a few hours it is a good idea to build up to this in the weeks or days leading up to the event, as leaving your baby for the first time can be difficult for you both.

Get your Little One used to the person who'll be caring for them, whether that's your partner, mum, a friend or a babysitter.

20-30 minutes
Why not pop to the shops, go for a walk or have coffee with a friend a few times?

1 hour
Leave your baby for an hour or so when you feel ready and see how that goes.

A few hours
A few days before your event, leave your baby for a few hours; maybe you could use the time to care for yourself and have a bit of relaxation.

A day
You've built up to leaving your baby gradually so they aren't faced with you suddenly disappearing for ages. You can now feel confident they'll be well cared for and content until you get back.

Childcare Choices

In Your Home:
Nanny or nanny share
Mother's help
Au pair
Relative

Away from Home:
Nanny share
Childminder
Nursery
Relative
Crèche

Choosing the right childcare for your family

The most important aspect in choosing childcare is to trust yourself and your own judgement. Reputation, friends' and neighbours' experiences and Ofsted reports may be helpful, but if it doesn't feel like it's the option for you, keep on looking. You'll never feel happy and confident leaving your baby with someone or somewhere you have doubts about. Very good childcare may be offered in far from state-of-the-art buildings, and not so good in a more impressive space – it is the quality of care and the people offering the care that are crucial for your baby's happiness. Be fussy, ask lots of questions and look around. Choose what feels right for you, and not whatever relatives, friends or neighbours are doing – every family is different. Childcare is expensive and it is important you feel you are getting the quality care your Little One needs, somewhere they will be happy and have their practical and emotional needs met.

Checklist for Childcare Away from Home

❏ Do the children look happy or a bit lost?

❏ What is the ratio of adults to babies?

❏ Are the staff playing with the children? Is there lots of fun and laughter?

❏ Do they ask you questions about your baby? Do they know your baby's name?

❏ Will your baby be expected to fit into their routines or is there some flexibility?

❏ Do the children have some choice and are they treated with respect?

❏ Is it clean and comfortable? Does your baby look engaged during your visit? Are there nice toys to play with and new experiences to have?

Checklist for Childcare in Your Home

❏ Is there a rapport between your baby and the interviewee?

❏ Do they seem genuinely fond of children?

❏ Do they ask questions about your baby and how you do things?

❏ Are they flexible, with a good sense of humour, or do they seem to have a strict way they like to do things?

❏ Do you feel warmly towards them? Would you be happy having them in your home and that they'd become part of your family?

❏ If you were in your baby's shoes, would you want them looking after you?

There have always been working mothers. A child benefits from a working mother in lots of ways, and it works really well for many families. If it doesn't work out for you, you can always change things. Just do what is right for you and your baby.

Returning to work

Many mothers go back to work during their Little One's first or second year, and managing this can be challenging and be a cause of anxiety for many reasons. Your baby takes their cue from you, so being positive and your usual self when you start to leave your baby with an alternative caregiver will help them feel relaxed and secure.

If you can, begin with short absences; just build up to being away for a few hours when you feel ready. Even with a young baby, have a little 'bye for now' routine. If your baby is awake, don't just disappear or sneak off when your baby is not looking, as it is important your baby has a sense of trust and security about your leaving. Babies do like the familiar, so any little ritual that shows you're going but will soon be back will help them understand what's happening and be confident that you are coming back. It's best if you don't linger, though; just saying a cheery goodbye (even if that's not how you are feeling on the inside – it can be very upsetting to leave your baby) and letting the caregiver start to play with, sing or talk to your baby will help them settle down better once you are gone. If your Little One does get upset about you leaving, cuddles and a little bit of sympathy won't spoil them at all. It is understandable that your baby is upset, but as long as someone else is there to meet their emotional and physical needs, all will be well.

Five Tips to Having a Happy Baby When You Leave for Work

1 **Be calm**
Your baby will pick up on your anxiety. It's important you feel confident your baby is in safe hands.

2 **Be positive**
You and whoever is caring for your baby can talk encouragingly about the lovely new experiences your baby will be having.

3 **Take your time**
Don't show you are in a hurry. Give your baby cuddles they need to feel secure.

4 **Have a mini-goodbye routine**
Keep goodbyes positive and fun, with a little phrase, a song, a little wave that you do each day that is calm and reassuring without making a song and dance about it.

5 **Don't sneak off**
Unless your baby is asleep, don't be tempted to go when they aren't looking.

In the weeks before you return to work, get your baby used to their childcare by gradually increasing the time they are separated from you. First you might want to stay with them, then leave them for just half an hour, then an hour, then a few hours. Don't be rushed or expect too much of yourself and your baby. If you can, give yourself enough time to let your baby set the pace so when you return to work you can feel confident they will be happy and safe. It may feel that you are having to share them when you only have a few precious weeks left before your maternity leave ends, but the more you can do to help your baby feel secure with their new carer, the better it will be for everyone.

If your baby is upset about the separation, don't let anyone laugh, mock or mimic them when they get tearful. They need gentle reassurance and empathy, and for their feelings to be acknowledged. It may make you feel guilty about leaving your baby, but as long as they are going to be well cared for and you are doing everything to make it a positive experience for them, you are doing everything you can. Be positive and resist the urge to be over the top when you go – your Little One will take their cue from you, so the calmer you can be, the better. That little 'bye-bye' waving routine will help to minimise distress for both of you. Your baby's carer can really help by distracting them with a game, toy or new activity while you swiftly leave them to have a lovely fun day. (You can always phone to reassure yourself that your Little One is settled and happy. A good carer will always be happy to update you on how your baby is and what they are up to.)

When you get back from work, give them lots of cuddles and be responsive. Be prepared that they might be upset when they see you. Some babies do cry when they see their mum; it's not because they've missed you the whole time or don't want to see you. It is just them processing that change in their lives.

Breastfeeding and Returning to Work

You can continue breastfeeding when you return to work if you want to.

1 **Express and freeze**
In the weeks before your return to work, express breast milk and freeze it in clearly labelled bags.

2 **Choose childcare close to work**
If you want to continue breastfeeding for some time, choosing childcare that is near your work will give you the opportunity to breastfeed as you drop them off and immediately when you pick them up. You might also be able to stop by at lunchtime to give your LO a feed, but do make sure you get food yourself – you'll need it!

3 **Give them yummy food**
If your Little One is over five months and is already enjoying solid foods, then they could continue enjoying their food topped up with expressed breast milk when necessary.

4 **Express milk at work**
Ask your employer if they have a lactation room where you can express milk in comfort and privacy (no one should have to express or feed their baby in the toilets!). You'll also need a fridge where you can store the milk, and a cooler bag with ice packs for taking it with you.

5 **Moving on from breastfeeding**

If your baby is under one year they will need to go on to first- or second-stage formula. There's no need for follow-on milk; if your LO is over a year old they can go on to cows' milk. You've done an amazing job breastfeeding and should give yourself a pat on the back.

If you want to stop breastfeeding ahead of going back to work, please look at the advice in Chapter 1 on how gradually to stop breastfeeding and move your baby on to a bottle or a cup. If you need to switch over to formula milk or need any advice on bottle feeding, have a look at Chapter 2 as well.

Parents who work can be very firmly attached to their Little Ones, and whether you are leaving them by choice or necessity mums have often worked outside the home and raised happy, well-adjusted children. Your Little One understanding that both women and men work can be a very positive thing to have in their lives and also gives them the opportunity for new experiences as well.

Some women do feel a bit low on confidence about returning to work after having a baby. In my experience, working mothers have so much to offer. If anyone can be strong, flexible, adaptable, organised and able to think on their feet, it is the parents of very young children. You can be proud of all you've achieved during your time at home with your new baby. The understanding you now have of how to meet another human being's practical and emotional needs doesn't just make you a wonderful parent but someone of high value in any workforce, because you know that you get the best out of people when they feel secure and happy, no matter how old they are. You've been your own boss during maternity leave and have faced completely new situations and developed a new skill set at an incredible pace. As your family continues to grow and adapt past your baby's first year, continue to follow your baby's lead, trust yourself and do what is right for you to have a happy baby and a happy family.

The Happy Baby A–Z of Practical Care

Baby-proofing

As Eeyore says, 'They're funny things, Accidents. You never have them till you're having them.' There is no such thing as having a baby-proof home, but there is a lot you can do to keep your baby as safe as possible at home.

It is worth getting into good safety habits before the baby is born, and thinking about routines when using the cooker and hob or making hot drinks. Ensure there are no trailing flexes and have the kettle to the back of the work surface so that it is out of reach. Look at any glass on doors and windows and use some shatter-proofing from the DIY store or, if you are replacing any windows, use toughened glass.

Fit a carbon monoxide alarm if you have gas or open fires, as it will alert you to any leakage of this very dangerous and harmful gas. Ensure you have a working smoke detector on every floor of your home, and test they are working once a week. Your local fire service will often advise and fit detectors for you. Have an escape route worked out in case of fire and practise this with the family. Keep your front and back door keys handy, but not in the door for security.

Have a 'baby safety day' before your Little One starts to be mobile. Look around your home for possible hazards room by room and try to minimise the risks by looking for hard-edged fittings like fire surrounds or sitting room and bedroom furniture that could hurt your baby if they fell on it. Drawers and cupboards need to be secure and not able to trap little fingers. Child-locks for cupboards and safety catches and plugs for power sockets are widely available and inexpensive, as are toilet seat locks and protective edges for the corners on furniture.

All cleaning materials and products need to be out of reach and locked away in the bathroom or under the sink. All medicines, especially everyday stuff such as paracetamol, aspirin, ibuprofen, iron supplements, vitamins and the contraceptive pill, all need to be in a high, lockable cupboard. Babies and children find shiny tablets and capsules irresistible and can't tell the difference between them and sweets. When visiting older relatives who may have their medicines to hand, watch your crawling baby or they might eat some while no one is looking.

Gates, room-dividers, playpens and travel cots can be really useful to prevent a crawling baby or toddler getting into spaces that are dangerous, such as the kitchen. It is worth investing in the sort of equipment that suits your accommodation and lifestyle to keep your baby contained when you need to, but babies should never be left unsupervised.

In the garden or park, be aware of possible hazards from plants and trees that may be poisonous, or equipment your baby could climb and fall off. At home, put in safety measures around furniture like bookcases that would make a perfect step or ladder for your curious Little One to scale new heights. Babies falling off a bed is a common accident, so be aware that your baby may suddenly roll over and off the bed with no warning. Once they start to crawl, bottom-shuffle or pull themselves up to standing and cruising along the furniture, all babies get a few bumps, and we can't prevent everything – but we can ensure a soft landing whenever possible. Try to be one step ahead of your Little One's development, as they have the curiosity and the stamina, as well as the determination, to explore their world and get into everything. That's their job; yours is to facilitate this as safely as possible.

Bathing

Bath water needs to be tepid and not too hot – remember to put cold water in first, then hot, to prevent patches of scalding hot water not being mixed in properly. It's a good idea to top and tail your baby every day (washing their face with just water and then their bottom with a tiny amount of gentle baby soap). Give them a bath three to four times a week, in a baby bath to start with, and once they can sit well and are splashing about, in the bath tub with a non-slip safety bath mat. Never leave your baby alone in the bath, even when they can sit up well. If the phone rings, let it, or take the baby with you. Some days babies will get really grubby (especially if there has been a poo explosion in their nappy!); other times you'll do them no harm by leaving a bath until tomorrow.

You can use your lap or the changing mat for dressing and nappy-changing. If it's possible it helps if there are two people the first few times you give your baby a bath, just for a helping hand while you're learning, as babies are rather 'slippery when wet' and you have to hold a new baby in the bath the whole time. It can be great fun, and it's a nice time to talk and sing to your baby and enjoy this time together.

Bathtime Essentials

Get everything to hand before you start to bath your baby.
Never leave your baby alone in the bath, even for a few seconds.

Baby bath or bowl
Cotton pads or cotton wool
Baby shampoo (use just a dot)
Baby soap or gentle soap (only use water for their face)
Clean clothes
Nappy
Warm fluffy bath towel
Baby moisturiser

If you remove the nappy just before gently lowering your Little
One into their baby bath, it's less likely they will have an accident. Start by dipping a fresh cotton pad in clean water and
squeezing out the excess water before cleaning your baby's
eyes and nose outwards. Use a fresh cotton pad for each eye.
Many babies have sticky eyes which persist on and off during
their first year, as tear ducts block easily; no need to worry
about this, it seldom bothers the baby. Use more cotton pads
to clean the face, especially neck creases, as milk trickles into
these and can make the neck sore. If this happens after bath
time, gently apply some of the cream you use on your baby's
bottom to heal soreness, then use a greasy product like bottom
butter or petroleum jelly to prevent it happening again. Wash
the rest of the face and behind the ears with the cotton pads,
but don't go into the ear. If you are using baby soap choose
mild baby soap that is gentle. If your baby isn't very keen on
having their hair washed in the bathtub, you can keep your
baby wrapped in a lovely fluffy warm towel and hold them over
the baby bath gently, pouring the water over their head, using

a dot of baby shampoo and then rinsing it off. Hair-washing needs to be done gently but swiftly, as tolerance can be short lived in this position for both of you. Wet the skin and wash the upper body, arms and underarms and then the lower body, the bottom, legs and feet.

If you have a baby boy there is no need to try and draw the foreskin back at all. The foreskin will only be ready from about four to six years, and sometimes later. Trying to draw the foreskin back can cause trauma, so just wash generally in that area.

If you have a little girl just wash generally around the vagina. I know sometimes parents think they have to wash inside the lips of the vagina as there is often a whitish look to the labia, but this is normal.

When your baby is all lovely and clean with that amazing baby smell, wrap them in a warm towel and gently dry them all over. Apply some cream to their body or, if they have dry skin, try using an emollient as this will help to keep the skin moisturised. If your baby develops a rash or seems to be having a reaction, stop using any product and ask your health professional for advice.

Bedding

Whether your baby is in a crib, a pram or a cot, babies should always sleep on their backs with their feet touching the bottom so their toes touch the end. Covers should be no higher than your Little One's shoulders and tucked in securely so the covers can't slip over their head. Never use a duvet, quilt or pillow for a baby, and in very hot weather your baby may only need a sheet or a muslin. It is better to have layers of blankets and sheets that you can add to or take away so you can easily and safely adjust your Little One's temperature.

In the winter months your baby will need two layers, and on chilly days a little cardigan as well when indoors. When going outside they'll need a hat and outer clothing with layers of blankets or sheets. Don't overdo the clothes and layers, and use how you feel yourself as a guide to whether you need an extra warm top or just a few light layers to keep out the cold. If you fold a blanket, remember that counts as two layers. Having a universal all-weather blanket that is suitable for use in a pram, buggy, car seat or bike seat can be very useful.

Birthmarks

Strawberry nevus

A painless and harmless birthmark not present at birth, but one or several can appear a few days after birth. They are often a small raised red spot that grows rapidly, and are produced from the extensive development of blood vessels. Although they grow rapidly, they then remain fixed at that size during the first year. Later, from 18 months to 2 years old or sometimes later, they subside, usually breaking up when a little whitish light area appears within the nevus and it then disappears altogether.

Haemangioma

Often similar in appearance to a strawberry nevus but more deeply situated, reddish/blueish and spongy. This birthmark is a mass of tissue filled with blood vessels. If in the nappy area it can be affected by the baby's wee and poo, and can sometimes bleed a little. This calls for frequent nappy changes and a protective layer of a nappy rash product. Your doctor may refer you to a specialist to assess and monitor this birthmark and to offer treatment if needed.

Port wine

Purple or reddish birthmark made up of dilated blood vessels, often seen on the face; they vary in size and shape. There are now treatments available on the NHS and your doctor can refer you to a specialist.

Pigmented nevus (moles)

Blackish and dark brown birthmarks. These pigmented patches are caused by clusters of pigment cells and can be sited anywhere on the skin, either singly or in clusters. They darken in the sun.

Blue spot

Blueish marks on the buttocks and/or lower back. These are seen in babies of Asian, African and Afro-Caribbean origin.

Café-au-lait

Light brown like milky coffee, hence the name. Occasionally the colour is a darker or blueish brown. If there are lots of these marks your doctor will note this and refer you for a specialist opinion if needed.

Bladder problems

It is quite common for mums to experience bladder problems (like a little bit of wee slipping out if you laugh or sneeze). The National Health Service offers a trained women's physiotherapist to help with this. Your health visitor or doctor can refer you and give you some pelvic floor exercises that will help tone things up a bit down there after giving birth. You usually get a leaflet on this in hospital or from your midwife or health visitor as well. If you are experiencing any problems, do tell someone; your six- to eight-week postnatal check-up with your doctor could also be a good opportunity to mention this or any other physical or emotional issues.

Blocked ducts

You may notice a small tender lump in your breast that could indicate a blocked duct. Try massaging the breast or using the warmth from a covered hot water bottle or warmed pad to help to disperse it. You may find this works best if you gently massage the breast to unblock the duct while you are in the bath or shower. This is best done after a feed; a good feed will help to empty the affected breast and clear the blockage. If a blocked duct does not clear it may lead to mastitis, so ask your health visitor or doctor for further advice at the earliest opportunity.

Bumps

If your baby takes a tumble and cries straight away, chances are that it is a bit of a shock but soothing cuddles may be all that's needed. If your Little One gets a raised egg-shaped swelling, then it's best to improvise an ice pack, using crushed ice or frozen peas in a plastic bag wrapped in a clean tea towel or muslin, to reduce swelling. If the baby was knocked out or has sustained an injury and is bleeding, stem the blood flow straight away and then you must get your baby examined as a precaution, even if they seem all right.

Burping

Winding or burping your Little One seems to dominate the early days and weeks. If you hold your baby in an upright position and gently rub their back, holding the head for support and gently moving them forward and then back, this often releases the wind. Some parents find that popping their Little One over their shoulder gives more relief and gets wind up, but there is no need to spend ages as babies tend to burp when they need to.

Chairs (baby)

Baby chairs, bouncers and seats are fine to use if they are safety-approved, but should always be on the floor and never on a high surface like a table or kitchen counter because your baby could fall or bounce off. Babies should never be left unattended in their high chair or seat. In a high chair, always use the safety straps. If you are in a restaurant or café and the high chair doesn't have straps, it is helpful to keep a pair of safety reins in your change bag to use instead.

Choking

Ensure small objects such as buttons and coins are kept well out of your baby's reach. Small round foods like whole cherry tomatoes and grapes should always be chopped in half to prevent choking. Be aware of ribbons and ties on baby's clothing, and toys which your baby could tear off and swallow or get wrapped around their neck. It is really good to go to a Parents' First Aid course in your area and get all the basics just in case.

Cleft palate

Sometimes a baby is born with a cleft lip or palate or both. The hospital will refer your baby to a specialist for treatment to repair the cleft. You can contact the Cleft Lip and Palate Association (CLAPA), which supports parents and provides information and advice as well as practical equipment like specialist teats and bottles so you can feed your baby. Contact them on 0207 8334883 or email info@clapa.com.

Colic

Colic, which literally means 'pain', is very uncomfortable for many babies and can be a source of anguish for you too. It is upsetting to see (and hear) your baby crying with colic; they go red in the face, get distressed and angry, draw their knees up, arch their backs and sometimes try to push off you with their feet and seem like they are trying to jump out of your arms (now is a good time to try the Happy Baby Up-Down Technique in Chapter 3).

Why do they do this? It's all part of their digestive system adjusting to life outside of the womb. Now their bodies have to work really hard to digest all their milk and as their tummy (which is only the size of their tiny clenched fist) gets full, they can feel very uncomfortable (just think of how uncomfortable you can feel when you've eaten too much). Colic is usually a short-lived spasm, but your Little One will have no comprehension of what is happening to them and won't know it will soon pass.

The best thing you can do for your baby is to stay as calm as you can and keep on going. It will be you who makes the real difference to how your baby feels. You can help them by soothing them with soft words, singing, giving them cuddles and lots of sympathy. It's not your fault your baby has colic, though it can sometimes feel like they suddenly don't like you – focus your mind on the calming technique you prefer to use, take a deep breath in and breathe out slowly; your stillness will go a long way towards calming your baby and help reduce your levels of anxiety, too.

There are colic remedies available on prescription from your doctor, and your health visitor can advise you on products which you can also buy at the pharmacy. Some simeticone products can help to relieve trapped wind, and can be used from the early days by giving a measured dose using the dropper before feeds – you'll find the dropper comes with the bottle, and instructions for the dosage are marked on it. A simeticone product takes 48 hours to work fully and it will not provide instant relief. It may be a couple of days or so before you see any results. In many babies there may be no improvement at all. After three or four days, if you don't see any improvement after giving the simeticone product, then stop giving it to them altogether. Never use more than one product at a time.

You can use gripe water from six to eight weeks. This product should provide immediate relief for colic and wind. One way to use gripe water is in just a little previously boiled and then cooled water (15–30 ml). It may be given in a sterilised plastic 5 ml spoon or in a little bottle.

Try only one product at a time and follow the instructions carefully. A pharmacist is often a great source of information on what's available to use. All babies are different in how they respond to colic remedies: some respond quite quickly and others hardly at all. You may find it is the comforting technique you use that gives the most relief to your baby, so keep an open mind and trust yourself to find the best method for you.

Cradle cap

A dry scaly condition of the scalp with hard, very dry and flaky scales that is very stubborn to treat. Gently rub in a little olive oil and shampoo off a few hours later (e.g. leave on overnight and shampoo in the morning). There are products on the market as well from the pharmacy, but try the olive oil first as the specialist products are costly and may not be effective for your Little One. You need to keep on treating and being very gentle with rubbing in the olive oil until the cradle cap starts to retreat. It seems to be very persistent in some babies while others are never affected, so watch out and nip it in the bud early on.

Dry lips and dehydration

If your baby has dry lips with little vertical lines instead of moist plump lips, they are dehydrated. When you see this they really need to have a feed; afterwards you will notice that their lips plump up again. This applies to everyone and you may notice it in yourself and others when they are dehydrated and need fluids.

Dry skin and eczema

It is common for babies to have patches of dry skin, and it's worth using sensitive skin products for washing their clothes, and using mild products for your baby's skin. Use only water and mild baby soap at bathtime. Avoid baby bath products as they can be drying. If you feel there is a problem, ask your health visitor or doctor to check your Little One's skin and give you advice on suitable products. Often there will be a specialist skin clinic for babies and children at your local baby clinic or hospital if you want an expert opinion and tailored treatment.

If your baby has eczema you will need advice from a medical skin specialist on how best to care for and treat your baby's skin.

Engorged breasts

You may experience engorgement in the week after birth. It is caused by the build-up of large quantities of breast milk, and sometimes by the increased blood flow to the breast. You may notice swelling and tenderness, that the breasts are too firm or feel tight, heavy and swollen and have a shiny appearance. Ask for help from your midwife immediately. If you aren't breastfeeding then sometimes wearing a tighter-fitting bra can help with the swollen, heavy feeling. You could discuss with your doctor any need for medication.

If you are breastfeeding then it will be frequent feeding that is usually most effective for relieving and clearing engorged breasts. Try to ensure the baby is in a good position and well latched on so they can get a really good feed and help to clear the breast of milk. Feed your baby every two to three hours. Gently massaging the breast in a downwards motion from the top of the breast towards the nipple, and applying a cloth-covered ice pack in between feeds may help to reduce the swelling. Keep warm, drink plenty of fluids and talk to your doctor about pain-relief medication.

Enlarged breasts (in your baby)

Your newborn baby boy or girl may have enlarged breasts which you suddenly notice when bathing or rubbing in skin cream. This happens when hormones transfer from you to your baby in the womb. They will resolve on their own in a few weeks and no treatment is necessary.

Expressing breast milk (EBM)

You can express breast milk either by hand or by using a hand or electric pump so your baby can get their milk from a sterilised bottle, cup or spoon rather than at the breast for a feed.

It is usually preferable to feed your baby at the breast and not to express milk in the early days but it may be something you want to do for a short time if you are experiencing sore nipples or you are separated from your baby. You may not be able to meet all your baby's milk needs through EBM alone but it can be a useful supplement alongside breastfeeding or for babies who are in a special care baby unit.

Breastfed babies need to get milk from both breasts as often as possible to establish and increase the supply of breast milk with frequent sucking. It is very unlikely that a mother can express the same amount of milk for her baby that feeding at the breast delivers, so unless there are special circumstances, like the baby being in a special care unit, I would advise that you feed from the breasts for the first two weeks or so to get the milk supply established.

If a baby is premature or poorly and is in a special care unit, a mum has no other choice than to use EBM if they are not allowed to put the baby to the breast. Whatever your circumstances are, expressing breast milk is hard work.

It often gives you flexibility, but some women find it draining, and you will need even more sustenance to both express and also breastfeed.

EBM can be really handy to have in the fridge when your baby is demanding huge amounts of milk in the night; it gives your breasts a rest, and if your partner takes over it'll give you a rest, too. Expressing milk does mean extra washing and sterilising of bottles and equipment (this is often a good job for your partner to take on; have a look at Chapter 2 to find out how to sterilise bottles and equipment). Many mums find that expressing after a feed works best. This milk can either be chilled in the fridge for up to 48 hours or frozen for up to three months for later use.

Pumps can be bought at the pharmacy, and some breastfeeding organisations lend out pumps, usually for a small charge, as electric pumps are expensive.

There are many pumps on the market but the important thing to remember is that they must be sterilised before each use and you will need to follow the instructions for correct assembly and usage. This is a job your partner could take responsibility for, as the pump needs to be 'built' before each use, and it is much better to be handed the pump sterilised, assembled and ready to go. Even if you prefer to express whilst your partner is at work, they could always get it ready for you before they go in the morning.

Eyes (sticky)

Many babies have recurring sticky eyes, which in nearly all cases are not harmful and can be cleaned by using cooled boiled water and cotton wool pads. Use one stroke from the inner aspect of the eye outwards. Be very gentle and repeat for each eye if needed, using a fresh cotton pad each time. If you are concerned, talk to your doctor for advice on how best to treat your baby.

Eyes (vision)

Your baby's pupils react to light from birth. The doctor will check your baby's eyes, especially for the red reflex to ensure they don't have a cataract. This needs to be detected at the earliest opportunity, as early treatment is vital. Some babies follow a face and they look at the light in a window from about the first week of life, and stare for a prolonged time at fairly everyday objects. You may notice this and wonder what they find fascinating about the wallpaper or whatever the object that is captivating them.

Fever (baby)

A fever for a baby is a high temperature over 38°C (101°F). Seek medical attention if your baby is under three months old and has a temperature. Also note if they have any other signs of being unwell such as floppiness and drowsiness. (See 'Illness', below, on how to count up the symptoms.)

Fever (mums)

Some breastfeeding mums experience a raised temperature, hot and cold sweats, aches and pains and generally feeling unwell, with flu-like symptoms. A raised temperature indicates that you have a fever. A normal temperature is around 37°C. If your temperature is over 39°C you should seek medical attention and advice from a doctor.

Fontanelle and shape of the head

The fontanelle or soft spot which allows your baby's head to grow is checked for size and position, and the head shape is noted by your health visitor, midwife or doctor. The measurement of the circumference of the head may also be taken and recorded. Many babies have differently shaped heads caused by their delivery, and these can take some time to settle. There may also be some bumps and lumps on one or even both sides of the head; these resolve on their own but your health visitor should keep an eye on them over the coming weeks, and your doctor should take a look at the six-week check.

Haemorrhoids and constipation

Constipation and haemorrhoids affect many mums, and may have been a problem for you while you were pregnant. Haemorrhoids, often called piles, are swollen and enlarged veins in or around the anus. They can be very sore and itchy and very uncomfortable, and you may have a feeling of lumpiness or that your bowel still feels full even just after you've had a poo. You may pass a little blood when having a poo, especially if you are constipated, which often happens in the days after you've given birth. Tell your midwife or doctor if there is blood. You may need a laxative like Lactulose to soften your poo if you have constipation, and a health professional or pharmacist can advise on preparations to treat the haemorrhoids as well.

An ice pack may ease the pain and reduce swelling. You can fill an unused condom with cold water and freeze it to make a small ice pack that you can press against the sore area around the anus. Fibre in your diet and drinking water more frequently will help get things back to normal. You can take action to prevent constipation by having vegetable soup, fruit and vegetables as well as wholemeal bread in your diet as soon as you start eating again after delivery. Do ask for help as soon as you can, as both constipation and haemorrhoids are treatable and you needn't carry on in silence if problems persist. I know it can feel embarrassing but it's an everyday part of the job for health professionals and it is something a lot of new mothers experience.

Hearing

All babies in the UK are screened at birth to ensure they have normal hearing responses, either in hospital or by your health visitor when she visits you at home. A very small number of babies have a single ear or both ears hearing problem, and early detection means they can get treatment from their first weeks, which significantly helps their development.

Hiccups

You may have noticed your Little One hiccupping in the womb. There is a structure in the body called the diaphragm, and it is this that separates the chest from the abdomen. It is the diaphragm that is involved in hiccups. Most babies have small bouts of hiccups which don't usually bother them and will soon pass; they are nothing to worry about.

Hips

Both of your baby's hips will be checked by a paediatrician at birth, at the six-week check with your doctor, and then at the seven- to nine-month check by your health visitor. If there is any cause for concern, your baby will be referred to a paediatric specialist.

Illness (minor)

When your Little One is poorly it's such an anxious time. Babies and children under five get, on average, a new infection every four weeks or so. This is to be expected and many will be minor infections you can cope with yourself with care and lots of cuddles and sympathy. Breastfeeding has the wonderful bonus of protecting your baby from infections, and if you breastfeed your baby you may find they get fewer or no infections during this time.

When your baby is unwell it may be helpful to count up the symptoms so you have a clearer picture of whether to seek medical help.

If your baby has a raised temperature (normal is 37°C, so a digital ear thermometer or strip thermometer you place on the body to read may be a good investment). Seek medical attention if your baby is under three months old and has a temperature over 38°C (101°F). If you notice any symptoms alongside a high temperature, such as a cough, runny nose, diarrhoea (more than eight loose poos in 24 hours), listlessness, being drowsy or floppy, or unusual levels of irritability, distress and pain, then get them checked over by a doctor.

If your baby has a couple of these symptoms but seems cheerful most of the time and it's a runny nose with a cough, then it may be a teething cough that you can manage very well – but if there are several symptoms and you are concerned, act quickly to see your doctor. You can ask for advice over the phone if you just want to confirm your own thinking that it's a minor cough or cold, but if you think your Little One is unwell and suffering or has a high temperature then you have a right to be seen quickly.

Immunisations

Parents, quite rightly, often have lots of questions about why their baby needs to have injections as part of universal immunisation. My answer is that more than any medical development in the last 50 to 60 years, it is immunisation that has meant today's children are protected from deadly diseases and survive infancy and childhood to become healthy adults. Before immunisation children were often seriously ill and died from common childhood illnesses like polio, tetanus and diphtheria.

Some babies are also offered the BCG jab to protect against TB if you have a living close relative who had TB in the past, or if you live in an urban area like London.

During my early nursing career in the 1970s I nursed children with measles who had brain damage and died as a result of this horrible disease. I know parents worry about vaccinations, but they really are the best way to protect your Little One. We would not be human if we didn't feel a pang for our babies during their injections, as no parent wants their baby to feel pain and discomfort, but it is short lived and your baby will be smiling again within minutes.

A severe reaction to immunisation is very, very rare in babies. They are able to take immunisation in their stride when an adult might have some reactions. After an immunisation you might find your baby is a bit fractious for a day or two, and sometimes the injection site is reddened and sore or a lump develops which gives the baby no pain as such but sometimes takes several weeks to go. Some babies have a raised temperature for a day after immunisation; if this happens you can ask your pharmacist for paracetamol oral medication, which is for use only after immunisation for babies from two months old.

Immunisations during Your Baby's First Year*

Two months (three injections)

1 First dose of 5-in-1 (DTaP/IPV/Hib) vaccine for diphtheria, tetanus, whooping cough (pertussis), polio and Haemophilus influenzae type b (Hib) to prevent pneumonia and meningitis

2 First dose of pneumococcal (PCV) vaccine

3 First dose of rotavirus vaccine

Three months (three injections)

1 Second dose of 5-in-1 (DTaP/IPV/Hib) vaccine

2 Meningitis C

3 Second dose of rotavirus vaccine

Four months (two injections)

1 Third dose of 5-in-1 (DTaP/IPV/Hib) vaccine

2 Second dose of pneumococcal (PCV) vaccine

Between 12 and 13 months (three injections)

1 Fourth dose of Hib and second dose of Meningitis C booster given as a single injection

2 Single injection against measles, mumps and rubella (MMR)

3 Third dose of pneumococcal (PCV) vaccine

* Immunisation programmes do change. Check with your doctor for up-to-date information.

Iron deficiency

Anaemia can be a problem for many women, especially in the months following the birth of their baby. Many women lose quite a substantial amount of blood during and following labour. You can check by looking at the lining of your eye: if it is very pale pink or grey-pink, you may well be anaemic and may need to take an iron supplement (red pink is the normal colour). Talk to your midwife or health visitor and have your haemoglobin checked with your doctor if needed, and get advice on what would be the best iron supplement for you to take.

Jaundice

Jaundice is seen in about half of all newborn babies. It is caused by the build-up of bilirubin (a chemical waste product) and shows as a yellowing of the skin and mucous membranes. The urine may appear darker, and poos may also be dark instead of yellow. If you are breastfeeding, do keep an eye on this as breastfeeding can help to clear jaundice. Your midwife will keep an eye on your baby until the jaundice has cleared. If your baby still has jaundice when they reach two weeks old, your midwife, health visitor or doctor will continue to check and monitor them and may test them for levels of bilirubin in their blood, as this would need further treatment in hospital.

Leaking milk

Leaking varies enormously among women: some mums find a crying baby (not always their own) causes leaking and can't leave the house without breast pads; other women have only a little leak now and then. Most women do need to use breast pads inserted in their bra to cope with leaking between feeds in the first months of breastfeeding, as this is when milk production is highest.

When there have been some hours between feeds, leaking is often copious and the first feed of the morning may soak your clothes whilst you are feeding from the first side, so it can be helpful to insert a muslin into your nightdress or top to mop up the milk if you haven't had the chance to put on your bra and a breast pad yet.

A little consolation for all this dampness is that you are producing lots of milk for your baby. You'll find that when weaning starts and you start to reduce the number of times you feed a day, you'll leak less and may not need to wear breast pads any more.

Mastitis

Mastitis can be a mild or severe inflammation of the breast and sometimes can cause fever and vomiting. If the breasts are painful and swollen and/or hot and red, you may have mastitis. Seek medical advice as soon as you notice the symptoms, especially if you have flu-like symptoms and are feeling hot and cold with achy joints and feeling generally unwell. Your doctor may prescribe some antibiotics if the mastitis has become infected, and also ibuprofen to help with the pain and inflammation. Only take medication as instructed by your health practitioner.

Drink lots of fluids and try using warm packs, or sometimes an ice pack can help, or even a small quantity of frozen peas in a plastic bag wrapped in a clean tea towel or muslin (remember not to eat the peas later on, though you could label them and refreeze for medicinal use again).

Do keep feeding the baby if you can, and check the position for breastfeeding and how the baby latches on to ensure you're going to be as comfortable as possible. (Revisit the Latching Techniques and positioning advice in Chapter 1 to double-check.)

Meningitis

Meningitis vaccines give excellent protection but can't prevent all forms of meningitis and septicaemia. Not every baby gets all the symptoms listed below, and be aware that they can appear in any order.

In babies the symptoms to look for are:
- a tense or bulging soft spot on the head
- high temperature
- baby is very sleepy, drowsy or unable to wake up
- baby makes unusual grunting sounds
- vomiting or refusing to feed
- breathing fast or having difficulty breathing
- irritable when picked up with a high-pitched or moaning cry
- blotching skin, getting paler or turning blue
- extreme shivering
- a stiff body with jerky movements, or else floppy and lifeless
- 'pin-prick' rash, marks or purple bruising
- pain/irritability as a result of muscle ache or severe limb or joint pain

- diarrhoea (sometimes)
- cold hands and feet.

If you are concerned, do the Tumbler Test: Press a clear glass tumbler firmly against the baby's rash. If you can see the marks clearly through the glass, seek urgent medical help immediately. If you are worried, call the Meningitis Research Foundation Helpline on 080 8800 3344

Milk spots (milia)

These are nothing to do with breast or formula milk. They are blocked pores that look like little spots of milk on the skin; they are very common in newborn babies. There is no need to treat these and you will notice that when your Little One is hot and bothered or crying they seem to glow like beacons, but when they are very calm or sleeping the spots almost disappear.

Nails (cutting)

When your baby is calm, curl their tiny fingers over one of yours to hold them steady and, using round-end baby scissors, give their nails a trim. If your baby doesn't like having their nails cut you could do it when they are sleeping. New babies' nails grow very fast and do need to be clipped once or twice a week so they don't scratch themselves too much.

Nappy change

Many parents prefer to change their baby on a change mat on the floor to prevent them rolling off. If you are changing them on a high surface like a bed or a changing table it is important always to be in touching distance to prevent them falling. Have everything to hand before you start: a fresh nappy and some cotton wool and water or wipes. If you are out and about it is good to have a spare set of clothes in your change bag for those inevitable mishaps. Some parents use cotton wool and tepid water in the early days to take extra care of their newborn baby's skin, but if you want to use wipes from the off for convenience that's fine. You can choose from disposable or reusable nappies – use whatever is best for you. There are plenty of brands to choose from for both types of nappies, and some local councils offer a cash incentive for using the cloth ones.

When changing your baby's nappy, girls should be cleaned from front to back to prevent germs getting into the vagina. On boys there is no need to pull back the foreskin, but do clean around the testicles and penis to keep their skin free from irritation. Many parents chat and sing to their baby to keep them calm and turn what seems like a never-ending messy task into having a bit of fun together. Without even thinking about it you'll be connecting with your baby and helping their speech and language development, too.

You need to change your baby's nappy frequently. In the early days you can expect to change around 10–12 nappies a day. When they get to around three to four months old this often drops to around 6–8 nappy changes per day. Frequent changing helps to prevent nappy rash, and it's a good habit to smear a protective layer of bottom butter or petroleum jelly on your baby's bottom.

Nappy rash

The best way to prevent nappy rash is to change your baby's nappy frequently and always thoroughly cleanse them of wee and poo so there's nothing left against the skin. Applying a layer of nappy cream, bottom butter or petroleum jelly on their bottom at every nappy change helps to protect the surface of your baby's soft skin from irritation. Babies often enjoy a bit of nappy-free time and the fresh air on the skin helps to keep them free from nappy rash.

Almost all babies do get nappy rash at some time, and swift treatment usually clears it up quickly. Nappy rash is caused by your baby's wee and poo irritating the surface of their sensitive skin, as well as by rubbing or chafing and possibly by a particular soap, detergent or bath product. If your baby has nappy rash there will red patches on their bottom, or the whole area may be red and raw-looking. The skin might be hot to the touch or have spots and blisters. If your baby has nappy rash, ask your health visitor or pharmacist to recommend a nappy rash cream. If the rash persists you may need a prescribed cream from your health visitor or doctor, and to get your baby checked for signs of thrush. If your baby has thrush the nappy rash creams won't work, as this is a fungal condition and you might also notice a white coating on baby's tongue, which will also need a prescription from a health professional to clear.

When babies are teething they often get an alkaline wee that burns the skin. You may notice tiny little red spots over the nappy area, which are small burns and are often mistaken for nappy rash. You can also help to prevent this with nappy-free time and using a greasy barrier layer of bottom butter or petroleum jelly on their bottom.

Sometimes babies get a pin-prick rash over their legs, arms and body, but if it is not in the nappy area it may be a reaction to washing products. Try using a different product and see if the rash goes or improves. Only use washing powder that is mild, and very gentle bathing products. Avoid the strong laundry powders, some bio- and non-bio detergents and fabric softeners, which often irritate babies' skin.

Nipples (cracked)

If your nipples are very sore and applying expressed breast milk or gel is not sufficient, then you may need to get a prescription for cream to heal the nipples. Any cream you use will need to be washed off before feeding the baby so they are fiddly and more time-consuming than using gel or hind milk. But sometimes if you use a cream for just 24 hours and let plenty of air get to the breasts, the nipple will heal a lot faster.

If you are suffering, using a cream to heal faster is well worth the bother, and much better in the long run than feeding on a very sore breast. Apply the cream in a thick layer, then wipe off with damp cotton wool before you feed your baby. I know this can be a real pain during night feeds, but do make sure it's all gone, as the baby should not ingest any of the cream.

While the nipple is healing you may want to breastfeed on only one side and express milk from the sore breast, just until it is comfortable to feed again.

If you are diagnosed with thrush, then not only will you need to finish any course of treatment to clear the infection but the baby will need to take oral medication as well.

Nipples (sore)

Having sore or painful nipples is probably the most frequently experienced problem women have when breastfeeding. In the first week it can be the result of your baby first learning to feed and your milk coming in, and it can be a toe-curling experience.

When your baby first starts to suck it may be painful for the first few seconds. If the pain persists, check the position of your baby – they may be sucking on the end of the nipple and not getting the big mouthful of breast they get when correctly attached (revisit the Latching Technique section in Chapter 1). If this happens, slip your little finger in at the corner of their mouth and break the suction. Adjust your position and try using a pillow if you want to (even if you are out and about, there are little travel cushions you can slip into the change bag to make life easier when feeding in public). Raise the baby up and bring them up to the breast. Check they are nose to nipple and ensure they have an open mouth coming from below the breast to latch on, getting as much of the brown area of the nipple into their mouth as possible and having a good seal, not a 'gappy' one, and keeping the nose clear from obstruction.

When they have finished, squeeze out some hind milk and gently rub it into the nipple to help soothe and protect it. Using breastfeeding gels before and after feeding may also help make you more comfortable. Also, don't over-wash the breasts as this may actually be a cause of soreness.

Period (baby)

Sometimes a baby girl has a little 'show' of blood from the vagina that is caused by hormones that transferred from mum to baby in the womb. This usually resolves naturally and is very short lived, though it feels alarming at the time. Let your doctor and health visitor know if this happens.

Periods (mum)

After the birth of your baby your menstrual cycle may take some months to return and may be different from your pre-pregnancy cycle. It is important to know that breastfeeding does *not* prevent pregnancy, as even if your period has not yet returned you may still get pregnant.

During breastfeeding women often have only a light period or no period at all. As feeding becomes less frequent or you give up breastfeeding, many women find that their menstrual cycle is irregular or that they experience a much heavier flow than before pregnancy. If you have any concerns about menstruation talk to your doctor, Family Planning or Sexual Health Clinic for advice and contraceptive care.

Posseting (throwing up milk)

Posseting is common in most babies and is an old-fashioned word that we use for babies who bring up little bits of vomit after feeding or sometimes even during a feed. It is normal for babies to posset because, as they burp, often some partly digested feed comes up. Many babies will be experiencing symptoms of colic as well as posseting from birth to six months, so it is no wonder it makes many parents feel anxious.

Posseting is nothing to worry about unless you think it is affecting your baby's weight gain and well-being.

You cannot stop your baby being sick but you can help them by feeding frequently (usually every two to three hours); raising the head end of their crib by placing a folded blanket or muslin underneath their mattress so your baby can rest in a more upright position; and giving your baby the opportunity to be on their tummy during regular supervised 'Tummy Time'. Once they can sit up with support, being upright may help lessen their vomiting reflex. Once babies start to wean and are having solid food and spend more of their day in an upright position, most parents notice they posset less or not at all.

Postnatal depression

It is very common to be a bit down at some point following the birth of your baby. If you think about the overwhelming change and responsibilities you now have, it is unsurprising that so many new mums have some feelings of depression or are just feeling a bit flat and out of sync. Postnatal depression can range from feeling a little down and over-anxious to severe anxiety and depression that require medical supervision. Your health visitor will usually do a quiz with you called the Edinburgh Postnatal Depression Scale (EPDS – see pages 93–5). The aim of this is to see if you are having feelings of anxiety or depression and to give you the opportunity to talk about your feelings and get further support if you need it. Your health visitor may suggest options for the help that is available for you. If you don't feel like you can talk to your health visitor, then your doctor will also be able to offer help and support. (See Chapter 4 for further information.)

Reflexes

Grasp reflex – holds on to finger tightly
Moro reflex – startled reaction
Rooting and sucking reflexes – baby roots around to find the nipple and then sucks vigorously

Reflux (GORD)

A small number of babies have Gastro-Oesophageal Reflux Disease (GORD) when acid from the stomach leaks out and back up into the oesophagus. Sometimes this is confused with posseting, which is very common in new babies, who frequently posset or vomit up some of their milk feed during or after a feed. In babies, reflux occurs when the milk feed 'flows back' up the baby's food pipe and is either projectile-vomited or, in the case of silent reflux, is regurgitated back up in the oesophagus and swallowed again.

Reflux requires a professional medical diagnosis and treatment as the acid reflux may cause inflammation of your baby's food pipe and affect their weight gain. If you think your baby has reflux and are worried they are not gaining weight and are in pain and distress, ask for a referral to a paediatrician to investigate and treat if needed.

Scratches

Babies are always scratching themselves and their nails can be like tiny daggers, scratching you as well. Invest in some round-end baby scissors for cutting their nails each week. Babies do heal very quickly, so an angry, red scratch in the morning may fade by the same evening. You can pop a tiny smear of healing cream on if you want to.

Skin to skin

Put your naked baby (with or without nappy) against your bare chest or tummy and hold them close. Relax and enjoy your baby. Skin-to-skin contact as soon as possible after birth is beneficial for babies, mums and dads – it is a very special feeling and provides comfort, warmth and security for your Little One.

Sterilising

As well as bottles, teats and formula milk, you'll need a steriliser and a bottle brush for washing – one that is never used for general washing-up. Before you put anything in the steriliser you will always need to:

1 Wash the bottles and teats thoroughly, as it is not possible to sterilise something that is not clean first;

2 Wash in warm soapy water very thoroughly;

3 Rinse in cold water afterwards to remove all soap residue.

Follow your steriliser's manufacturers' instructions.

Stitches or tearing

Your body has done some very hard work in labour and delivery and you may have had stitches or a tear that needs time to heal. Your midwife in hospital and then at home will be the best person to discuss any concerns you have. If you are experiencing pain, discomfort or are concerned about the stitches, it is worth getting them properly checked by your midwife or doctor.

Many stitches are dissolvable but some stubbornly refuse to dissolve and cause discomfort, itching and soreness. Your midwife can check the healing for you and remove them if they have done their job and you've healed, even though the stitches may not have dissolved. Many women find that two to three drops of tea tree oil in a daily bath can help soothe things if you've had tearing and/or stitches. If you don't have a bath tub, applying very gentle pressure with warm (not hot) water from a hand-held shower can also be beneficial in soothing the perineal area, which you can dry with the warm setting on your hairdryer, as rubbing with a towel may only add to your discomfort. Wearing soft cotton knickers will not only be more comfortable but help keep the area as dry as possible.

Some women find they are still bleeding or have a dark red spotting of blood for several days before it darkens to brown and then to a straw-coloured discharge. This can be hard to deal with; finding the time to care for yourself when you have a new baby to take care of, combined with feeling fed up with the whole process, is a challenge for many mums after giving birth. Some women find it makes them feel unattractive or have some feelings of revulsion; this should not last for long, and if it persists for several weeks or months then do discuss these issues with your health visitor, doctor or the sexual health team at your local clinic.

Stork marks

This is a whimsical term for red marks caused during delivery on a baby's face and head. They can form a broken ring over the eyes and skull, and happen while the baby passes through the birth canal. They fade with time and your midwife may point them out to you so you can check they are going.

Sun safety

Babies under six months should be kept out of the heat of the day, especially between 11 am and 3 pm when the sun is at its hottest. Babies should have no longer than 20 minutes exposed to direct sunlight in very hot and sunny weather. Use sunblock and dress your baby in a layer of cool cotton. Cover your Little One with a muslin or very lightweight sun-safe blanket if they are in their pram. Ensure your baby has sufficient fluids and feeds frequently. In hot weather your baby may like a drink of cooled boiled water from a sterilised bottle that has been kept in a chiller bag. Once your baby has sucked on the teat it will no longer be sterile and can't be used again, so if they haven't finished it throw the contents away. If your baby is over six months old you could give them a drink of bottled water if the seal is unbroken.

Swaddling

Swaddling is wrapping your baby in a light cloth such as a large muslin square or swaddling cloth before popping them down to sleep in their crib or pram. I prefer to leave their arms and hands free in a half swaddle, as most babies like to have their hands free to suck. A half swaddle still gives your baby the womb-like warmth and security without restricting them, and often helps babies to fall asleep gently. If your Little One really doesn't like swaddling after a few goes, don't worry, swaddling isn't for them. (See Chapter 3 for instructions on how to do the Happy Baby Half Swaddle.)

Testicles (enlarged and swollen)

Baby boys can have extra fluid in one or often both testicles. This usually disperses gradually over several months and your doctor will check for this at the six-week check, and review and refer if necessary to a specialist doctor.

Testicles (undescended)

Your baby boy may have been born with one or both testicles undescended (a doctor will note this during baby's first medical exam if they do not feel two testicles in the scrotum). It is not a cause for concern, and you may have noticed that even descended testicles move about a bit anyway. Your doctor will feel the scrotum again at the six-week check to see if the testicles have made their way down. Often testicles move down naturally all on their own in the first three to six months. If they have not moved down by the seven- to nine-month check with your health visitor, they may refer you to a paediatric surgeon for their opinion. If you have any concerns, talk to your doctor or health visitor – you don't have to wait until the checks.

Thrush (you and your baby)

If you or your baby has thrush then you will both need treatment, as it easily passes back and forth between mother and baby unless the infection is treated for both of you until it clears. If your baby has oral thrush they might have a white coating on their tongue or white patches elsewhere in the mouth that do not rub off easily like a milk coating does. To check, give your baby an ounce or so of cooled boiled water in a sterilised bottle. If the white area goes, it is not thrush, but if it is still there it may be thrush and will need treatment. You might notice your baby is reluctant to feed and stops feeding if their tongue feels sore.

It may be that you had vaginal thrush in pregnancy and it transferred to the baby during delivery. It makes sense to treat a baby with oral thrush and also to check for bottom thrush, and ensure that vaginal thrush is treated in you to break the cycle. Do not blame yourself or worry about this, as it is very common in babies and no reflection on you, and is easily treated. Your health visitor or doctor can give you a prescription.

Tongue-tie

Tongue-tie is when the frenulum, a short string-like membrane under the tongue, is tightly attached to the floor of the mouth rather than loosely attached. If your baby has trouble sticking out their tongue and it doesn't go past their gums, or pulls into a heart shape, they may be tongue-tied. If your baby latches on and feeds well, and is gaining weight, they may not need any treatment. However, if your baby finds latching difficult and is not feeding well, ask your health visitor or doctor about whether they think it would help to clip the frenulum.

Travel (car seats)

Strapping your baby into car seats and buggies is essential whether you travel by car or public transport. If you'd had a hospital birth you'll need a car seat to take your Little One home, and it is sensible to practise how to fit the car seat before your baby arrives so they can be safely strapped in for their first journey. The law requires all babies and children to use a safety car seat, and there are leaflets in your clinic or from road safety organisations that are useful when it comes to choosing the right one for your family.

Tummy button (umbilicus)

Your baby's umbilicus can become brittle and have dried blood on it which is tough to remove, or be oozing fluid and become sticky, or bleed a little. All of these are quite normal. To ensure good healing, clean the tummy button two to three times a day using a fresh cotton pad soaked in cooled boiled water and then squeezed out. Wipe gently but firmly around the tummy button to keep it clean. Usually the cord drops off between four and eight days after birth, but sometimes they stay a little longer. The sight of it does bother a lot of parents, as it looks a bit alarming, but there is no feeling in the umbilical cord and even though the baby may flinch when it is cleaned it is because the water is cold; there are no nerves and therefore no feeling in the cord. If there is a little tag of flesh protruding this may be a granuloma – your health visitor will discuss treatment and care of this, which is quite common and not serious.

Urine (baby)

Your baby's wee should be clear and colourless. They should have at least six wet nappies a day. Note if their urine is ever dark (in newborn babies this is a sign of jaundice) and let your midwife or health visitor know.

Walkers

Baby walkers are not advisable, as there are many accidents caused each year by their use and they actually delay mobility as babies are not using the right muscles for natural growth and development. Spending time together doing fun things on the play mat or doing an activity like baby yoga or baby massage are lovely ways to have fun with your baby, relax and nurture their development. A few minutes every day right from the start of supervised time on the play mat and then Tummy Time is time well spent rather than leaving your baby to their own devices in a walker or jumperoo. If you do want to use one, though, ten minutes a day of supervised time is enough.

Winding

Winding helps to minimise colic and should be done in a gentle manner. Some babies posset a little during winding, so have a muslin or cloth handy.

Wind is a build-up of gases in the stomach. With all the feeding your baby does there is inevitably a lot of wind in their tummy, which causes gripe pains. By winding and burping your baby you are helping them to bring up some of that gas so they feel more relaxed and happier.

1. Grey/blue top lip
2. Grimacing smile
3. Stretching and pushing away from you

Winding Techniques

1 Sitting upright

Sitting your baby in an upright position on your knee helps release the wind in the tummy. There is no need to vigorously pat and bang your baby's back; a gentle circular rubbing movement combined with tilting the baby forwards and backwards will often do the trick.

Winding Technique One

1. Sit your baby upright on your knee.
2. Hold them under the chin between your thumb and forefinger.
3. Gently rub the small of their back in small circles with the flat of your other hand.

2 Over the shoulder

You may find that once your baby is fully fed, putting your Little One over your shoulder may be a good position to get some wind up.

Winding Technique Two

1. Hold your baby securely with the flat of your palm on the small of their back.
2. Rest your baby's body against your chest with their head and neck over your shoulder.
3. Bring up your other hand and use the flat of your palm to rub their back in a gentle circular motion.

3 Outstretched legs

Winding Technique Three

1. Rest your baby on your outstretched legs with their feet pressing on your stomach.
2. Hold each ankle and gently bend their legs and move their feet towards their tummy.
3. Gently rock their feet back down, then repeat a few more times to help alleviate wind.

Acknowledgements

Thank you to our agent Piers Blofeld and Hannah MacDonald, who believed in our work. Helen Braid for her beautiful illustrations.

Never forgotten are the inspirational nurses and health visitors who shaped my practice with families – Patricia Wrennall, Désirée Knox Whyte, May Paulus and Daphne Claw. For ground-breaking work with children pioneered by Dr Mia Kellmer Pringle and Dr Mary Sheridan.

Special thanks to Catherine Powell, Anona Matthews and Susan Footner for being a listening ear and discussing ideas on children, health and education.

To Elizabeth Riddell for her love and support and for taking such good care of our LO. To wonderful friends Mark and Matt Beyer-Woodgate.

Huge hugs to the mums, dads and their babies who have been with us on this journey – Jake and Dulcie Alexander, Boglarka Apostolne Haui, Lucy Beeson, Fateha, Nazia and Abeda Begum, Pippa Best, Rachael Blair, Rhiann Bramwell, Elisabeth Buckley, Lucy Coward, Faye Draper, Emma Evans, Nazia Farookhi-Bailey, Boxa and Nicole Francis, Robin and Kelly Grace, Kelly Henderson, Rosie Lewis, Caroline Maher, Nicola MacKinnon, Rose Maguire, Emma Markiewicz, Dr Karen Osburn, Antonia and James Peck, Katie Pekacar, Emma and James Read, Katy Ross, Sarah and Christian Sandy, Georgina Thompson, Tia Wallace, Jillie and Luke

Willcock, Lucy Williams, Megan Worthington, Sally Wrennall-Montes, Laila Zaghari and Canon Father Guy Wilkinson and Reverend Lesley Bilinda and all the mums and babies at Monday morning group.

Biggest thanks of all are for Takbir and Ava Beeson-Uddin. With love
Sarah and Amy Beeson

Also by Sarah Beeson MBE

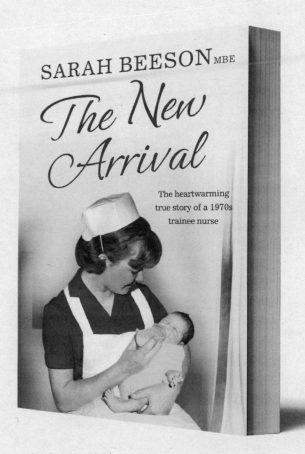

The heartwarming true story of a
1970s trainee nurse

1

It was 23 September 1969, already past nine o'clock in the morning. I was still sitting alone on the back seat of my father's blue Rover P4, waiting for my mother to emerge from the house. I impatiently kicked my white round-toed calf-length Mary Quant boots against the front passenger seat. After years of practice I could do this without scuffing either the seat or my well-worn but perfectly presentable boots. All the time I kept my eyes fixed on the open front door of Uplands, our *gentleman's country residence* – I was leaving as soon as my mother deigned to join me. 'Typical,' I muttered under my breath. I took my last long sniff of sea air and slowly counted to ten. My ears pricked at the distinct click of my mother's court shoes on the parquet floor; she was finally making her way down the hall and outside. Two steps behind her was Harold, my father's driver, carrying my battered old school trunk with the initials SH fading on the side. I watched icily as Mum unnecessarily oversaw Harold loading my trunk into the boot of the car before he opened her door and she slipped effortlessly onto the seat next to me. Neither of us said anything; we both sat straight backed with our knees together on either side of the back seat – my mother's handbag resting perfectly upright between us. Harold took up his place at the wheel and I felt my heart skip with excitement as he started the engine and we finally made our way down the quarter-of-a-mile driveway.

I watched idly through the window as we sped down the narrow country lanes to meet the seashore and the grey little town below. Llanelli whizzed past me, stonewashed modest houses, mothers pushing carriage-like prams, small vans delivering to butchers and greengrocers. It seemed such a small, small world. Too small for my mother. She sat day by day in the big house waiting for my father to return – one of the bosses at Thyssen's, he arrived home almost every night of the week with at least two dinner guests expecting to be served a three-course meal. Mum rarely complained. Also at the table, merrily sitting alongside Dad's international business associates, were my older brother and sister, William and Jane, the younger two, Bridget and Stephen, and often our school chums. Both children and adults consumed vast amounts of prawn cocktail and pink champagne off the custom-made boardroom-sized dining table. Dad would say to our dinner guests, 'You've got to be quick in this house,' as his gaggle of children lapped up our grub whether it was a curry, a Chinese or a roast.

This place was too small for me too; it wasn't my home, just the latest stop after a childhood of constantly moving to new towns and villages. Dad was a top civil engineer and we moved with him; so one year he would be working on the Dartford Tunnel and we were living it up in Sevenoaks. Next we'd moved into a house custom built by my dad, on the hilltop overlooking Loch Etive, while he built the new hydroelectric plant to supply electricity for the west coast of Scotland. I wouldn't miss this house; Scotland had been the beloved place of my childhood – it was there I made the transition from little girl to brooding teenager. Today, my only pang of regret was as the car went past the Chinese takeaway belonging to my best friend Sue's family. Of course the shutters were down at that time of the morning, but still I looked for her heart-shaped face in the upstairs window. She wasn't there.

Mum folded her hands, her long fingers cocooned in spotless white gloves which rested lightly in her lap. I peeked up at her and drank in her portrait. Her slender frame and long neck were enhanced by a cream polo-neck jumper, complete with matching coat and pillbox hat. Her hair was still naturally dark, though she was over fifty, and swept up into a glossy brown bun on the back of her head. She was perfectly made up with just a dash of powder on her pretty tanned nose, a sweep of grey shadow on her sparkly eyes and a smear of pink lipstick on her mouth – just right for this time of the morning. Beside her I was a pale-skinned dwarf. When standing, she towered a good eight inches above me, more in heels, which she usually wore. Apart from my obvious lack of height compared to the rest of my family, I took more after Dad on the inside too. Put together my brothers William and Stephen were like a pair of giant bookends. My sisters Jane and Bridget were tall and graceful like Mum. But though we all got into our fair share of scrapes, I was always the one to unintentionally rile my mother or be in hot water with the nuns at boarding school, as I shared my father's sense of fun, sometimes at the expense of what we *ought* to have been doing. I wished it was just me and him driving to London on one of our rare drives together.

I heard Mum sigh as Harold deviated from the main road down yet another narrow country lane – one of his so-called shortcuts that doubled the length of the journey. 'We won't be there till sunset at this rate,' she hissed.

It was the second thing she'd said to me all morning, the first being, 'Is that what you're wearing?' I'd come down to breakfast in my red suede miniskirt and black polo-neck top.

I was eager to be off and already wearing my three-quarter-length navy Reefer jacket with the brass buttons, my hair still wet and falling unfettered and uncut to my chest. I considered it a rhetorical question, and moodily helped myself to the toast, jam and a cup of tea which were all ready and waiting on the breakfast table.

Now the silence was broken Mum settled upon a topic for the journey – her incredulity at both my choice of career and location. 'All the money your father's spent on your education. You won't last two weeks.'

I didn't say anything in reply. I leaned forward and asked Harold if we could have the radio on. He tuned in to Radio One just for me. Mum huffed and opened up her square white leather handbag and to my relief took out her knitting. I was glad to hear the friendly familiar voice of Tony Blackburn on the car radio as he introduced The Archies, and soon the sound of 'Sugar, Sugar' filled the highly polished Rover.

But my mother had made her point and I couldn't help but think back to my last year at school – my secret study in the library. I kept going back and reading up on nursing. I had been pretty appalled at the life of a nurse too, and yet I felt so drawn to it. I wanted to make a difference in the world and to help people who needed care and compassion. When my grandfather had been very sick it had been me who sat with him, comforted and cared for him, not my brothers and sisters or even my parents, who had been uncomfortable around illness. It felt to me it was the right thing to do; it felt like it was my gift to him. But even my friends hadn't thought nursing a worthwhile ambition – nice privately educated young ladies weren't meant to do that sort of thing (unless you count my heroine Florence Nightingale, of course).

It wasn't until I was summoned to the headmistress's office that I made my final decision. She informed me, 'Sarah, I've put your name down for teacher training,' something nice respectable girls could do until they had babies. I found myself replying, 'Well, that's a surprise as I'm going to be a nurse,' and flouncing out of her office feeling as pleased as punch. As soon as I'd done my O-levels I went to do my Community Voluntary Service in a children's home in Wiltshire. I knew then that nursing was my calling. I'd completed my nursing application and accepted my place without consulting anyone. I'd not told my parents or even mentioned it to my siblings. My parents were horrified at my decision – here I was, 17 years old and going to be a student nurse in Hackney in the East End of London of all places. This life was not what anybody had in mind for Sarah Elizabeth Hill.

Ours was a happy, busy family, there was always something going on – Stephen accidentally setting fire to my father's wood or the farmer's pigs getting in and eating the precious crop of strawberries – but our parents had high expectations. Bridget my roommate was sitting her exams and Stephen wasn't even a teenager, yet William was studying civil engineering at university under duress and Jane was doing fashion at art college.

Why, I asked myself, was it suddenly necessary to be driven down by Harold with my mother as escort? After all, they'd been sending me on buses, trains and planes unaccompanied to boarding school from infancy. I decided it was all down to Mum's morbid curiosity, or most likely the hope that I'd take one look at the nurses' accommodation and hot foot it back to South Wales in Dad's chauffeur-driven car. Well, if that was the plan, my parents were going to find themselves disappointed.

The car finally edged its way down bustling Homerton High Street early that afternoon. There was a constant buzz of small delivery vans and buses going up and down. The pavements and the houses were narrow and greyish and rows and rows of small shop fronts made up the face of the high street. Harold pulled into the grounds of Hackney Hospital and parked next to the large circular lawn at the front of the nurses' home. It towered above us; six storeys high of 1930s' sandy-grey brick – relentlessly flat and institutional looking. I looked up at the neatly stacked uniform windows in the plain block; I couldn't wait to know which one would belong to me.

'Is this it?' said my mother in disbelief. 'What a dreadful place; I don't think your father will like you living in this sort of neighbourhood.'

I jumped out of the car, eager to stretch my legs and find my room. Harold was already taking my trunk out of the boot. 'Just pop it in the entrance, please, Harold. I'll take it from there,' I instructed. He silently went ahead and disappeared into the building. Mum was still in the car. She wound down the window slowly. I went round to her side of the car and popped my head in. 'I'll be fine from here. You get off,' I tried to insist in what I thought was a casual but confident manner.

'No, I want to make sure you'll be all right,' she said, opening the car door as I stumbled back.

'All right,' I said, stalking off to the entrance, passing Harold on his way out of the building with my mother hot on my heels.

I pushed my way through the heavy double doors and stepped into the large whitewashed hall. It was plain, yet purposeful. Heavily curtained windows proceeded straight and tall down the length of the black-and-white tiled corridor. At the end, a staircase curved off and up into the heart of the building. I saw Harold had placed my trunk under the wooden table that stood on a faded though spotless rug in the hallway. The table, bathed in shadowy light, was made welcoming by a vase of white carnations. This was the entrance to my new life – I was home.

'It's very clean,' said my mother, running a gloved finger over the table. 'Like a hospital. Smells like one too,' she added with a twitch of distaste. She couldn't be doing with hospitals or sick people; they made her feel uncomfortable.

'You'd better get going, Mum. You want to be back in time for Harold to pick up Dad from work.'

'I thought I'd see your room, take you into town for a nice lunch. Make sure you're properly fed.'

'I'll be fine,' I insisted. I knew Mum was worried, that she was trying to be kind, but I just wanted to get on with things – I have always hated long goodbyes.

She looked into my face, searching for some hint of whether she should insist I return home with her right now. 'If only you were at a nice hospital in the West End or Grosvenor Square, near your father's head office.'

'I want to be here. I will be fine. Please don't worry.'

Mum turned and then hesitated. 'If you're sure …'

'I am,' I said, stepping forward and giving her a brief hug.

I could see Harold through the pane of glass in the big front door. The engine was running – he knew the score.

'If you're sure,' she repeated, and this time it wasn't a question. I smiled and gave her a single nod of the head as I opened the double doors for her and she walked steadfastly back to the Rover.

She paused once again as her hand reached for the door handle. I gave a little wave of encouragement from the front step of the nurses' home and to my relief Harold appeared at her elbow to open the car door and she slipped elegantly inside. 'Safe journey,' I called.

'I'll write,' she called back through the open window as the car pulled off back down the drive towards the gates. I saw her quickly winding it back up again as they found themselves once more heading towards Homerton High Street.

Back in the nurses' home I made my way gingerly down the corridor, passing cleaners sweeping and polishing, and nurses hurrying in and out; no one took any notice of me – everyone had a job to do and soon I would too. I had to head directly to Home Sister's room to report for duty. I remembered from my interview in the summer that it was just to the left of the main entrance. I almost skipped as I trotted past the half-open door of the reading room, glancing at the white caps peeking up over the tops of chintzy sofas – but I did a double take when I spotted uncovered greased-back hair looming over the tops of the armchairs. Hang on a minute – men, men are allowed in the nurses' home, I said to myself. I guessed this room wasn't really for reading and study but somewhere to meet up with your boyfriend. *NB!* I laughed quietly to myself. Just as well Mum hadn't accompanied me or I'd have never been shot of her; she hadn't put me in a convent boarding school for nothing.

Once in front of Home Sister's inner sanctum I took a deep breath and knocked on the door. I waited but there was no answer. I knocked again but still nothing. I thought I heard a noise from within, a soft shuffle and a clink. I hesitated and cast my eyes about. What was I to do? Where was I to go?

'You looking for Home Sister, pet?' I heard a voice behind me sing out down the corridor in a lyrical accent I'd never encountered before.

I turned round and saw a small nurse in a light blue dress and crisp white apron smiling at me, her hip resting against the wall. Her bright blue eyes crinkled up at the corners; she must have been at least forty. She had wild curly chestnut hair poking out from under her nurse's cap and red lipstick stained her plump little mouth. With two highly arched black eyebrows and a perfectly round blush on each of her white cheeks, she looked like a china doll. I thought make-up was forbidden.

'Yes, I was told to report to Home Sister on arrival.'

'Hill, is it?'

'Yes.'

'I'm Wade. Edie Wade. Home Sister is, shall we say, indisposed.' I looked blank. She softly chuckled and mimed taking a drink and then played the drunk wobbling about a bit and bumping into the wall. I stifled my laughter, placing my hand over my mouth. 'You should have come before lunch,' she told me.

'Oh, we didn't arrange a time.'

'You'll learn the right time soon enough. Come on, I'll show you to your room.'

'Thank you,' I replied rather meekly, my former confidence ebbing away a little at having already been shown to not know the score in front of a real nurse.

'Where are your bags?'

'My trunk is under the table in the hall.'

'Is it now? Well, I'll ask the porter to bring it up to you. You're on the fourth floor, room 17. You wouldn't want to heft it up all that way yourself. Follow me,' said Wade, tapping off down the corridor and springing up the stairs. My spirits lifted by her easy manner and dancing feet, I rushed after Wade, following her little black shoes as she did toe heel leads all the way to my room.

'I've only been here a week myself,' said Wade.

'You're a nurse already though, aren't you?'

'Not young enough to be a trainee, hey?'

'No, no, I meant ...'

'I'm only teasing you, pet. I've been a nurse off and on in-between bairns ever since I left the music halls. I'm here to do my midwifery.'

'You were in the music halls?' I asked, amazed and impressed.

'Ever since I was little girl. I've done a turn with Morecambe and Wise, not to mention Julie Andrews,' she told me, belting out 'The Hills are Alive with the Sound of Music'. I looked around, embarrassed and unsure of what to say next.

Wade took a key out of her pocket and unlocked the door before handing it over. It swung open to reveal a small rectangular cell lit by a single window. I stepped into my new room; it was simply furnished, just a single bed with neatly folded sheets and blankets resting on it, waiting for me to make it, a bare wooden chest that folded out into a desk and an empty cupboard. A hand basin stood in a little recess, with a mirror and vacant shelves above it waiting to be filled with my things. Apart from that there was only a laundry box which served as a seat. I walked over, removed the lid and peeked in.

'I keep bottles of booze in mine. It's the one place Home Sister won't scout them out,' snorted Wade. I smiled broadly. My room.

'There are no plugs in here so if you want to use a hair dryer or anything you'll have to make do with the hall socket. I'm just next door,' continued Wade. 'Have you eaten?'

'No,' I replied.

'Ah, come with me then, I'll show you the nurses' dining room – it's almost tea time. Home Sister normally rallies after a good strong cup of tea.'

I obediently followed Wade. There were already dozens of nurses sitting at round tables, which were covered in white table cloths with a place neatly laid out for each girl. I walked behind Wade to the counter. My eyes met with bowlfuls of pies, mash, sausages, chips, roasted meats, curry, rice, fish, bread rolls, soup, umpteen traditional puddings, jugs of custard, and pots of tea and coffee. It was tempting stodge and I vowed not to make a habit of eating it and looked penitently at the salad bar.

'What do you fancy, Hill?' she asked.

'What are you having?'

'My regular – sausage, eggs, bacon and a fried slice of bread with a cuppa.'

'I'll have the same. How much is that?' I asked, reaching into my pocket for my purse.

'You've forgotten it's "all in". Bed and board.'

'Oh, yes of course, how silly of me.'

'Come on, we'll eat up and then try our luck and see if Home Sister is ready to receive callers. You'll need your uniform pressed and ready before you see Matron at eight o'clock tomorrow morning. I've heard you're starting on the Infants Ward. It's nice there but watch out for that Sister Nivern, she's a right devil; you do not want to get on the wrong side of her,' Wade instructed me, as she heaped sausages on to my plate for tea.

At the thought of what Sister Nivern might have in store for the new girl, I almost lost my appetite.

Index